THE BEGINNERS GUIDE TO GUT HEALTH

UNLOCKING DIGESTIVE FREEDOM, WEIGHT WELLNESS, AND MENTAL CLARITY MADE EASY

CHRISTINA B. KISER

TABLE OF CONTENTS

INTRODUCTION

Eighteen years ago, I received a diagnosis that would change the course of my life: Hashimoto's disease. For nearly two decades, I wrestled with its array of symptoms, from debilitating fatigue to unexplained weight fluctuations. Despite endless medical appointments and treatments, relief seemed elusive. During one particularly challenging day, struggling to muster the energy to get out of bed, I realized I needed to take a different approach. That realization began my deep dive into gut health, a journey that transformed my health and rekindled my zest for life.

This book is born out of that personal journey. It's crafted to demystify the complex science of gut health, linking it directly to weight management, mental clarity, and an enriched sense of overall wellness. I know firsthand the frustration of wading through dense scientific articles and conflicting health advice. That's precisely why this guide has been crafted—to distill complex scientific concepts into clear, simplified language that seamlessly integrates into your daily life.

I understand the struggles many of you face—whether it's puzzling health symptoms, overwhelming fatigue, or the frustration of not feeling heard by your healthcare providers. This book is your ally and guide, offering a compassionate perspective from someone who has walked in similar shoes and found a path to better health through understanding and nurturing the gut.

Here, we'll explore the pivotal role of the gut in our health, the transformative power of probiotics, and the vital connection between our digestive system and mental well- being. You'll find clear, actionable advice on adjusting your diet, making lifestyle changes, and employing natural remedies to enhance your gut health. Each suggestion is backed by the latest studies and expert insights, ensuring you have reliable, scientifically accurate information.

Perhaps most importantly, this book promises to equip you with the knowledge and tools necessary to take control of your health journey. By understanding your gut's crucial role in your overall well-being, you can make informed decisions to improve your quality of life.

So, I invite you to join me with an open mind and a readiness to explore your body's potential to heal and thrive. Together, let's navigate this journey toward digestive freedom, weight wellness, and mental clarity. It's a path well worth traveling, and it starts right here, with the first step towards understanding and improving your gut health.

CHAPTER ONE

UNDERSTANDING YOUR GUT

D id you ever stop to think that right now, as you sit reading this, there's a whole civilization bustling inside you? Yes, trillions of microbes are hard at work. It's not science fiction—it's your gut microbiome, and it's a bigger deal than you might think. This chapter will unfold the secrets of this hidden world within you, revealing how this tiny ecosystem profoundly impacts your health, mood, and thought processes.

1.1 THE GUT MICROBIOME: A HIDDEN WORLD WITHIN YOU

Diverse Ecosystem

Imagine your gut as a vibrant city, teeming with trillions of microorganisms such as bacteria, fungi, viruses, and other tiny inhabitants. This diverse ecosystem functions like a dynamic urban environment, where the wellbeing of its microbial citizens is crucial for maintaining the city's overall health and efficiency. This diversity isn't just impressive—it's vital. Each microbe has a specific role that helps your body function optimally, from digesting food and producing vitamins to warding off harmful pathogens. The richness of this microbial diversity is a critical player in your overall health, acting much like an ecosystem capable of affecting everything from your digestion to your immune system.

Balance is Key

Imagine walking on a tightrope. You must maintain perfect balance to avoid falling. Similarly, the equilibrium among the various microbes in your gut is essential. When this balance is disrupted—say, more harmful bacteria take up residence over the beneficial ones—it can lead to many health issues, commonly known as dysbiosis. This imbalance can affect digestion and ripple out, influencing your immune response, weight, and mood. Maintaining this delicate balance is a critical aspect of your health. Factors like diet, stress, and antibiotics can tip this balance, sometimes with significant and lasting effects.

Impact of Lifestyle

Your lifestyle choices stand out in the drama that unfolds in your gut. Every meal you eat, every stressor you experience, and every medication you take is like sending a wave through this delicate ecosystem. For instance, a diet high in processed foods and sugars can feed the less beneficial bacteria, allowing them to overpower the beneficial ones. Similarly, chronic stress can alter your gut flora's composition and function, making you more susceptible to illness. Even antibiotics, while sometimes necessary, can act like a tornado sweeping through your gut, wiping out swathes of both good and bad bacteria, often leading to further health complications if not managed properly.

Foundational Health

Your gut microbiome is not just about digestion. It's the foundation upon which much of your health is built. An imbalance in your gut can lead to more than just stomach issues. It's linked to a range of severe health problems, including obesity, diabetes, and chronic inflammatory diseases. Think of your gut health as the bedrock of a building. If the foundation is weak, the entire structure is compromised. By taking care of your gut, you're not just avoiding gastrointestinal issues. You're potentially warding off various ailments and boosting your overall health.

Understanding this hidden world inside you is the first step towards harnessing its power for better health. As we explore the depths of your gut microbiome, remember that every small step you take—swapping a sugary snack for something more wholesome or taking a few minutes to destress—can profoundly impact this vibrant, bustling metropolis within you. It's about making choices that support the balance and diversity of your gut residents, ensuring they, in turn, can help you lead a healthier, happier life.

1.2 HOW YOUR GUT HEALTH AFFECTS YOUR WHOLE BODY

Let's talk about a superpower you might not know you possess— the extraordinary ability of your gut to influence far more than just your digestion. It's like discovering you have a secret room in your house that simultaneously controls the electricity, water, and security systems! The gut doesn't just help break down food. It's deeply intertwined with your entire body, affecting everything from how well you absorb nutrients to how effectively your immune system functions.

Consider nutrient absorption—your gut is where the magic happens. It's where your body retrieves the necessary vitamins, minerals, and energy from your food. When your gut health is on point, it's like a well-oiled machine, efficiently extracting every bit of goodness from the food, ensuring that your body gets all the nutrients it needs.

However, if your gut isn't in top shape, it's like having an inexperienced team handling the most vital operations of your business. You might eat a diet rich in all the good stuff, but without a healthy gut, your body might not reap the benefits, leading to nutrient deficiencies and all the troubles they bring.

Moving on to the immune system—your body's defense department—the gut also plays a critical role here. About 70% of your immune system is located in your gut. Think of your gut lining as the high-security wall that keeps out potential intruders. A healthy gut helps ensure this barrier remains impenetrable, allowing only the good guys (nutrients) in and keeping the bad guys (pathogens) out. However, if this barrier is compromised, it's like the gates of the castle being left open in a medieval battle. Invaders can quickly enter, leading to infections and increased vulnerability to illness.

Moreover, an unhealthy gut can lead to an overactive immune system that misfires, which can cause inflammation throughout the body—this isn't just a tiny skirmish. It's an all-out war where your body ends up fighting itself, leading to many autoimmune conditions.

Turning our attention to a topic that frequently challenges many—weight management—the gut microbiome acts as your body's economic advisor, influencing not only how your body stores fat and regulates blood glucose levels but also how it signals hunger or satiety. When the gut microbiome is out of balance, it's like following the advice of a misguided financial planner, leading to disarray in your metabolism. This imbalance can result in weight gain, diabetes, and other metabolic disorders, highlighting that successful weight management is not solely about counting calories or selecting the proper diet. It's fundamentally about nurturing a balanced, symbiotic relationship with the microbial community in your gut, ensuring your metabolism operates smoothly, just like that well-advised financial strategy. Therefore, managing your weight goes beyond the surface of dietary choices; it's deeply intertwined with maintaining the equilibrium of your gut's inhabitants.

Lastly, the gut acts as a protective barrier against external pathogens. A robust gut lining is like the body's ultimate bouncer, deciding who gets into the club and who doesn't. When this barrier is intact, it prevents harmful bacteria and toxins from entering the bloodstream. This is crucial because once these unwanted guests get past the gut lining, they can travel to other parts of the body and cause severe health issues. Keeping this barrier strong is one of the most effective ways to maintain health and prevent disease.

Through all these roles—nutrient absorption, immune function, metabolic regulation, and protective barrier—the gut has a systemic influence that extends across the entire body. Its health or dysfunction can set the tone for your overall health, much like how a conductor influences the performance of an orchestra. Ensuring your gut is healthy isn't just about avoiding bloating or discomfort. It's about tuning this complex system for optimal performance, enhancing every aspect of your health. So, the next time you think about eating that extra cake or skipping your probiotics, remember that the stakes are higher than you might think. Your gut is not just about digestion. It's the cornerstone of your health, silently and powerfully influencing your entire body's well-being.

1.3 SIGNS AND SYMPTOMS OF AN UNHEALTHY GUT

Let's get real about some of the distress signals your body might send you from the gut department. Have you ever had one of those days where it feels like your stomach is plotting a full-scale rebellion? We're talking about bloating that makes your jeans beg for mercy or gas that could rival a parade balloon. Yes, we've all been there, and though it might be a bit embarrassing or even comical at times, these symptoms are your body's way of waving a red flag that something's off with your gut health.

Chronic digestive issues such as bloating, gas, diarrhea, and constipation aren't just minor nuisances. They're significant indicators that your gut microbiome may be imbalanced. When this balance is disrupted, it can lead to a series of discomforts: bloating, diarrhea, and constipation. Each of these conditions makes daily life increasingly challenging. However, the impact on your gut extends well beyond merely processing food. It plays a pivotal role in your overall health, influencing much more than your digestive tract alone.

Moving beyond the belly, let's talk about some systemic symptoms. Have you ever noticed your skin freaking out with rashes or acne when your stomach is on the fritz? Or maybe you've felt like a battery running out of juice, struggling with fatigue that no amount of sleep can fix, or finding that your scales seem confused, showing weight fluctuations that make no sense? These can all be distress signals from your gut. When your gut is unhappy, it can lead to inflammation, which plays out in various ways, from your skin to your energy levels. It's like having a silent alarm system that impacts your entire body, signaling that the balance within your gut is causing more than just digestive upset.

Now, let's tread into the territory of mood fluctuations. Ever felt more anxious or down in the dumps than usual and couldn't figure out why? Emerging research is shining a light on the gut-brain connection, suggesting that an imbalanced gut can be a party pooper for your mental health, exacerbating symptoms of anxiety and depression. It's fascinating yet somewhat unsettling to think that the tiny microbes in your gut could affect your mood. They produce and influence neurotransmitters, like serotonin, which is critical in feeling good. If your gut is out of sorts, it might send mood-dampening signals to your brain, turning a sunny outlook into a series of cloudy days.

Lastly, if you're dealing with an autoimmune condition, it's worth considering the state of your gut health. Conditions like mine, Hashimoto's, can be linked to what's happening in your gut. An unhealthy gut can ramp up inflammation throughout your body, potentially triggering or exacerbating autoimmune responses. It's like having a spy inside your body's defense system, where the gut's skewed messages can lead to your body mistakenly turning on itself, resulting in autoimmune flare-ups.

Recognizing these signs and symptoms is crucial. They are not just inconveniences. They are your body's way of calling for help, suggesting it's time to pay attention to your gut health. Whether it's the bloating that disrupts your day, the fatigue that won't lift, or the unexplained mood swings, these signals are interconnected, pointing to the gut as a key player in your overall health scenario. By tuning into these signals, you can start making changes that improve your gut health and enhance your overall well- being, turning what feels like a body in rebellion into one in harmony.

1.4 THE GUT-BRAIN CONNECTION: HOW YOUR GUT INFLUENCES YOUR MOOD

Let's take a fascinating detour into the realm where neuroscience meets gastroenterology. Yes, it's a thing! This is about the gut-brain connection, a hot topic unraveling some intriguing insights into how your gut can play puppeteer to your brain's emotions. Before you brush this off as sci-fi material, let me assure you that it's all backed by science and incredibly relevant, especially when you feel like your mood swings are in the driver's seat.

Imagine there's a superhighway between your gut and your brain. This isn't a road filled with cars but messages zipping back and forth. This highway is known as the vagus nerve, one of the longest nerves in your body, which acts as a two-way communication setup. It's like having a direct phone line between your gut and brain. The brain sends signals about stress or anxiety to the gut, which can affect digestion and gut function. Conversely, your gut uses this line to return its status updates to the brain, influencing your mood and emotional well-being. This communication is pivotal, as it can mean feeling anxious or calm, foggy-brained or clear-headed.

Now, let's talk about the little workers in your gut: the bacteria. These tiny beings are like chemical factories, churning neurotransmitters such as serotonin and dopamine. You heard that correctly — gut bacteria make the same chemicals traditionally attributed to the brain. Serotonin is often called the 'feel-good' neurotransmitter because it can contribute to feelings of happiness and well-being. Surprisingly, much of your body's serotonin is produced in the gut. So, it stands to reason that if your gut is out of sorts, it might lead to a dip in serotonin production, leaving you feeling less than your best.

The plot thickens when considering how these gut microbes affect your body's stress response. If your gut microbiome is out of balance, it can seriously affect your body's ability to handle stress. It's like having a security system that is too sensitive, triggering false alarms at the slightest provocation. This high-stress response can lead to an increase in anxiety and depression symptoms, making it harder to cope with daily stressors. It's a vicious cycle: stress can disrupt the microbiome, and a disrupted microbiome can heighten stress response.

But here's the silver lining—by modulating your gut health through diet and lifestyle changes, you might find a powerful ally in the battle against mood disorders. This isn't about quick fixes. It's about making sustainable changes that nurture your gut flora.

For instance, a diet rich in fiber, probiotics, and whole foods can foster a robust microbiome, stabilizing your mood and enhancing mental clarity. Moreover, regular exercise and proper sleep can also significantly maintain a healthy gut-brain axis.

This burgeoning field of psychobiotics explores how diet and lifestyle modifications that improve gut health could be used as a novel approach to treating mood disorders. It's about using the knowledge of the gut-brain connection to our advantage, creating interventions that might help with symptoms of anxiety and depression through the gut rather than traditional medications alone. The therapeutic potential here is immense, highlighting a future where we might see dietary plans prescribed as part of treatment for mental health problems.

So, next time you're feeling down or overly stressed, consider that your gut might be trying to tell you something before you let it spiral. A tweak in your diet or a new approach to managing stress might be the key to a healthier gut and a happier, more balanced you. This understanding of the gut-brain connection underscores the profound interconnectivity of our bodies and emphasizes that sometimes, the answers to our health issues can be found in unexpected places.

1.5 PROBIOTICS AND PREBIOTICS: KEY PLAYERS IN GUT HEALTH

How about those unsung heroes of your gut health: probiotics and prebiotics? Imagine them as your gut's nurturing parents, where probiotics are the beneficial bacteria that make your gut their home, and prebiotics are the nourishing food that keeps these bacteria happy and thriving. Together, they form a dynamic duo Know as synbiotics, which can significantly boost your digestive health and beyond. Understanding these elements can be as transformative as discovering a hidden treasure in your backyard, promising health benefits.

Probiotics are like the friendly neighbors in your gut community, always ready to lend a helping hand. These live bacteria and yeasts are crucial for maintaining a healthy gut environment. They help break down food, absorb nutrients, and fight unwelcome pathogens. Think of them as your digestive system's peacekeepers. Their benefits don't just stop at digestion. Research suggests they play roles in bolstering your immune system and potentially improving skin health, and they could also play a role in elevating your mood. Those little critters could work full-time to keep your stomach and spirits high!

But these microscopic helpers need the proper sustenance to thrive, and that's where prebiotics come in. Prebiotics are dietary fibers that human enzymes cannot digest but are a feast for beneficial gut bacteria. These fibers are not just roughage but are found in foods like bananas, onions, garlic, leeks, asparagus, and many others. They are the power food for your probiotics, helping increase populations of healthy bacteria in your gut.

When probiotics and prebiotics combine, they create what we call synbiotics. This combination isn't just good, it's synergistic, meaning they work together to create a sum greater than their parts. Synbiotics ensure that the probiotics have the right environment to work effectively, enhancing overall gut health, supporting your immune system, and potentially boosting your mood.

Now, while you can get a good dose of these beneficial elements from foods, sometimes your diet might not meet your gut's needs, and this is where supplements come into play. The supplement aisle can be overwhelming, with countless options that claim to be the panacea for all gut issues. Here's where a bit of savvy comes in handy. Not all probiotics supplements are created equal. The key is to look for supplements that contain live and active cultures, and it's often recommended to choose products with multiple strains of bacteria, as each strain contributes differently to gut health. For prebiotics, focus on supplements that contain natural fibers like inulin or fructooligosaccharides. However, starting slowly with prebiotics is crucial to avoid any initial bloating or discomfort as your gut adjusts to its new residents.

As you navigate this overwhelming market, consider your specific needs. Are you looking to improve digestion, boost your immune system, or manage stress better? Understanding these can guide your choices, ensuring you bring home the right guests to your gut's ongoing block party. Remember, the goal is to create a balanced, thriving micro-community in your gut where everyone works together harmoniously.

Incorporating these superheroes of the gut world into your life doesn't have to be complicated. It can be as simple as swapping your morning bagel for a banana or adding asparagus to your dinner plate. Minor dietary tweaks can lead to significant health enhancements. It's about making conscious choices that delight your palate and feed your gut's best friends. And if you're stepping into the world of supplements, a chat with a healthcare provider can set you on the right path, ensuring that your journey towards a healthier gut is as smooth and effective as possible.

With every fiber-rich vegetable and every dose of a multi-strain probiotic, you are not just feeding your body. You are cultivating an ecosystem that, in return, supports every aspect of your health. So, the next time you sit down to plan your meals, or wander down the supplement aisle, think of yourself as both a gourmet chef and a savvy gardener who's not just eating for taste but nurturing a flourishing inner garden. Your gut—and, by extension, your whole body—will thank you for it.

CHAPTER TWO

COMMON GUT ISSUES DEMYSTIFIED

Have you ever had one of those days where your stomach feels like it's hosting a rock concert, complete with a mosh pit, in your intestines? If so, you're not alone, and it might not just be last night's questionable takeout to blame. One of the most common headliners in the world of gut health issues is Irritable Bowel Syndrome, popularly known as IBS. It's like the uninvited guest who crashes your internal party and refuses to leave. Let's dive into the nitty-gritty of IBS, stripping away the complexities and misconceptions to arm you with everything you need to take back control of your gut health.

2.1 DEMYSTIFYING IBS: WHAT YOU NEED TO KNOW

Prevalence and Impact

IBS is not just a minor inconvenience. It's a significant health concern affecting 10-15% of the global population. Imagine filling several football stadiums of sufferers, and you've just about got the picture. It's more common among us ladies, so it's high time we talk about it without hushed voices. Living with IBS can feel like being on a rollercoaster you never bought tickets for, impacting everything from your social life to your professional world. The unpredictability of flare-ups can cause anxiety and stress, which— spoiler alert— only makes the symptoms worse. It's a pesky loop that can significantly diminish one's quality of life.

Symptom Spectrum

The symptoms of IBS can vary from one person to another, ranging from mild annoyances to severe disruptions that can make you want to camp out near a restroom permanently. The classic hallmarks include abdominal pain, bloating, and a mix-up of bowel habits—some days you might experience constipation, other days diarrhea, or, if you're fortunate, a delightful combo of both. But here's the kicker: not everyone's experience with IBS is the same, and the triggers can be as individual as your morning coffee order. This variability is why managing IBS often feels like trying to solve a mystery wrapped in a riddle, wrapped in a tortilla of confusion.

Trigger Identification

Identifying what triggers your IBS is a game-changer. It's like becoming a detective in your own life, scrutinizing everything from your diet to your stress levels. Common culprits include certain foods (dairy and gluten), hormonal changes, medications, and, yes, stress. But here's a fun twist: sometimes, it's not just what you eat but how you eat—wolfing your meal while multitasking might stir up trouble in your gut. Recognizing these triggers isn't just about avoiding discomfort but empowering you to make choices that keep the peace internally.

Management Strategies

Now, on to the battle tactics! Managing IBS doesn't have to involve drastic measures. Sometimes, small lifestyle and diet adjustments can bring significant relief. Let's talk about diet first. Fiber is often hailed as a hero, but here's where it gets tricky. While soluble fiber (in foods like apples and oats) can be soothing, insoluble fiber (hello, bran) might trigger symptoms. It's about finding the right balance for your body. Then, there are probiotics. These good bacteria might help restore order in your gut's microbial community, reducing symptoms.

Stress management is another critical piece of the puzzle. Activities like yoga, meditation, and regular exercise can lower stress levels and improve gut function. It's like hitting two birds with one stone—calming your mind and soothing your gut.

Lastly, consider medication. Certain medications can help manage symptoms when lifestyle changes don't. But here's the deal: medication should complement, not substitute, lifestyle adjustments.

Reflective Section

To wrap up our chat on IBS, let's reflect a little. How often do you rush through meals? Do you find certain foods tend to send your stomach into a frenzy? Keeping a food and symptom diary can be an enlightening exercise. It helps you connect the dots between your eating and how you feel, providing clear insights to guide your dietary choices.

Plus, it's a great tool to bring to your healthcare provider, helping them tailor advice and treatment to your specific situation.

Navigating IBS is undeniably tricky, but minimizing its impact on your life is possible with the proper knowledge and strategies. By understanding the nature of the beast and how to tame it, you can move towards a life where your gut doesn't dictate your plans. So, let's keep this internal party under control, shall we? After all, life's too short to spend it in the bathroom.

2.2 LEAKY GUT SYNDROME EXPLAINED

Imagine your gut as a high-security fortress. This fortress is designed expertly to allow certain entities in and keep others out, maintaining a delicate balance crucial for your overall health. But what happens when the walls of this fortress start to crumble? This is essentially what occurs with leaky gut syndrome, a condition where the intestinal lining, or the "walls" of your gut, become more porous than usual. Usually, your intestinal lining acts as a control gate, allowing nutrients to pass into the bloodstream while blocking harmful substances. However, leaky gut syndrome compromises this lining, creating openings that let toxins, microbes, and undigested food particles slip into places they shouldn't be.

This increased intestinal permeability can be triggered by several factors, including excessive stress, poor diet (rich in processed foods, sugar, and alcohol), overuse of antibiotics, and inflammation. These triggers can disrupt the tight junctions, the strong bonds holding the intestinal cells together. When these junctions loosen, the gut's contents can leak into the surrounding area and bloodstream, setting off alarm bells throughout your body.

The systemic effects of leaky gut are far-reaching, linking to many health issues that might seem unrelated at first glance. When unwanted substances enter the bloodstream, the immune system kicks into high gear, recognizing them as foreign invaders and launching an attack. This response is good when it's pathogens you're fighting off, but when it's food particles or toxins, it leads to chronic inflammation. Over time, this persistent state of war can lead to more severe health problems such as autoimmune diseases, where the body, confused and overtaxed, begins attacking its tissues. Conditions like rheumatoid arthritis, lupus, Hashimoto's, and multiple sclerosis have been associated with this phenomenon. Additionally, allergies can become more pronounced as the body reacts to threatening substances.

Despite its significant impact, the leaky gut syndrome has been a point of contention within the medical community. Some experts question its validity as a distinct medical condition, arguing that increased intestinal permeability is a symptom or a contributing factor to other diseases rather than a standalone ailment. This debate has spurred various studies and research to uncover more about this mysterious condition. These studies strive to map out exactly how the intestinal barrier becomes compromised and the best ways to treat and manage it. The ongoing research is crucial as it sheds light on the intricate connections between gut health and overall well-being, pushing the boundaries of traditional medical paradigms.

Those looking to heal their gut and restore its rightful function should focus on diet and lifestyle changes that strengthen the intestinal barrier. Emphasizing a diet rich in whole, anti-inflammatory foods is a good start. Foods like bone broth, which is high in collagen, and fermented foods, rich in probiotics, can help fortify the gut lining and balance the microbiome. Anti-inflammatory foods such as leafy greens, fatty fish like salmon, and nuts are also beneficial. Besides dietary changes, reducing stress through mindfulness practices like yoga and meditation can significantly improve gut health.

Regular exercise, adequate sleep, and avoiding known irritants like non-steroidal anti-inflammatory drugs (NSAIDs) and excessive alcohol can also play pivotal roles in maintaining a robust intestinal lining.

Addressing leaky gut involves a holistic approach, focusing on what you eat and how you live. Adopting a lifestyle that supports gut integrity and reduces inflammation can reinforce your body's defenses and promote healing from within. This proactive approach helps manage, and potentially reverses the effects of, leaky gut syndrome, and enhances your overall health, enabling you to live a more vibrant, energetic life free from the discomforts of an unbalanced digestive system.

2.3 SIBO: SMALL INTESTINAL BACTERIAL OVERGROWTH

Imagine your small intestine as a quiet suburb suddenly overwhelmed by an unexpected, disorderly influx of bacteria. This is the essence of Small Intestinal Bacterial Overgrowth, or SIBO, where bacteria increase in the small intestine beyond normal levels. Unlike the colon, a bustling city of microbes, the small intestine should be a more serene environment with fewer bacterial residents. When this bacterial balance is disrupted and the small intestine's tranquility is invaded, a range of uncomfortable symptoms can emerge, including bloating, discomfort, and compromised nutrient absorption.

Now, why does this bacterial bash start in the first place? Several factors might roll out the welcome mat for these microbes. For instance, if the muscular activity of the small intestine—what sweeps bacteria down to the colon—slows down, bacteria seize the chance to multiply. Conditions like diabetes, scleroderma, or aging can slow these muscles. Sometimes, a single bout of food poisoning can damage nerves that control these muscles, leading to an open house for bacteria.

The symptoms of SIBO are not particularly unique, so it's often mistaken for other digestive disorders. Common complaints include nausea, bloating (usually severe), abdominal pain, diarrhea, or constipation (sometimes both, flipping back and forth), and in long-standing cases, weight loss and vitamin deficiencies due to malabsorption.

It's like your body is a garden hose with a kink. No matter how much water you put in, not enough comes out the other end, and the hose balloons up under pressure.

Diagnosing SIBO typically involves a breath test, which can feel like a high school science experiment. You drink a sugar solution and breathe into a bag at set intervals to measure levels of hydrogen and methane—gases produced by bacteria when they feast on sugars in the small intestine. Elevated levels of these gases can indicate SIBO. While this test isn't perfect, it's one of the best available tools without resorting to more invasive procedures.

When evicting these uninvited guests, treatment usually involves a combination of antibiotics and dietary changes. Antibiotics are like the police breaking up the party, effectively reducing bacterial overgrowth. However, the antibiotic choice, treatment duration, and potential for recurrence make this a tricky path. Adding to the complexity, different bacteria produce different gases, so treatment may be tailored depending on whether hydrogen or methane is more predominant in your breath test results.

On the dietary front, the approach is all about not feeding the crashers. A diet low in specific carbohydrates that bacteria love to feast on—known as the low-FODMAP Diet—can be beneficial. It's about avoiding foods that are high in fermentable sugars, which include, but aren't limited to, certain fruits, vegetables, dairy products, and grains. Think of it as not bringing snacks to the party - fewer bacteria hang around without food.

Now, let's consider the ongoing management and prevention of SIBO, which is crucial because these bacteria are keen to return like party crashers who had a great time.

Ensuring optimal gut motility is critical, keeping the digestive tract moving to avoid giving bacteria time to settle in and multiply. Sometimes, doctors prescribe prokinetics, which helps speed up digestion to keep things moving. It's like having bouncers in your gut, ensuring that bacteria move along to the colon, where they belong.

Moreover, regular retesting can be part of the management strategy. Especially if symptoms reoccur. It's a bit like checking your house after you've had intruders. You want to ensure everything is secure or, in the case of SIBO, that the bacteria haven't moved back in. Integrating a mindful eating routine— eating slowly, chewing thoroughly, and not overeating—also supports digestive health, which can prevent conditions that favor bacterial overgrowth.

Managing SIBO often requires a multifaceted approach that includes medication, dietary adjustments, and lifestyle changes to improve gut motility. It's about creating an environment in your small intestine that discourages bacterial overgrowth, all while ensuring that the rest of your digestive system is functioning optimally to prevent future issues. This proactive, comprehensive management strategy helps maintain a balanced, happy gut, minimizing the risk of these microbial party crashers returning.

2.4 THE IMPACT OF CANDIDA OVERGROWTH

Your gut is a vibrant ecosystem where a diverse community of microorganisms flourishes together. Candida, a typically harmless yeast that coexists peacefully in this environment, is one of these microorganisms. However, challenges emerge when Candida expands excessively, like a city grappling with overpopulation. This unchecked proliferation disrupts the gut's delicate balance, leading to a condition known as Candida overgrowth. It's not merely an issue of yeast abundance. It's the resultant imbalance that unsettles the gut's harmonious ecosystem.

Typically, Candida is a quiet neighbor, living in your digestive tract and on your skin without causing trouble. However, certain conditions can turn it into an unruly tenant, leading to overgrowth. Factors that commonly allow Candida to thrive include a diet high in sugar and refined carbohydrates, a weakened immune system, excessive alcohol consumption, and broad-spectrum antibiotics that indiscriminately kill beneficial and harmful bacteria.

The signs of Candida overgrowth can often be mistaken for other health issues, making it a medical chameleon. You may experience persistent fatigue, making your daily coffee seem like a drop in the ocean. Digestive problems such as bloating, constipation, or diarrhea can become frequent uninvited guests. Then there's the matter of recurrent yeast infections, fungal infections on the skin and nails, or oral thrush. These physical symptoms are often accompanied by difficulty concentrating, poor memory, mood swings, and irritability. It's as if Candida throws a wrench into the complex machinery of your body, causing gears to grind and sputter across various systems.

Addressing Candida overgrowth requires a holistic approach that looks beyond merely quelling symptoms. Diet plays a pivotal role here. Reducing your intake of sugars and refined carbs is like cutting off the fuel supply to an invading force, as Candida thrives on sugar. Emphasizing foods that foster a healthy gut environment can help restore balance. This includes incorporating plenty of fiber-rich vegetables, quality proteins, and healthy fats into your meals. Garlic, with its natural antifungal properties, can be a potent ally in your culinary arsenal against Candida. Coconut oil is another versatile player, rich in caprylic acid and known for its yeast-battling prowess.

Incorporating probiotics is crucial to replenishing and maintaining the army of good bacteria in your gut. Think of probiotics as reinforcements to restore order and support the local microbial community. Fermented foods like sauerkraut, kefir, and yogurt are not just nutritious additions to your diet. They're functional foods that help keep Candida in check by enhancing your gut's microbial diversity. Additionally, specific antifungal treatments, both natural and prescription-based, can be effective in directly combating an overgrowth. Herbs such as oregano, which contains the antifungal compound carvacrol, and extracts like grapefruit seed extract are popular natural remedies to fight yeast infections.

Preventing a recurrence of Candida overgrowth is about maintaining the balance and health of your gut's ecosystem over the long term. This involves consistent management of your diet and lifestyle factors that can predispose you to imbalances.

Regular consumption of probiotics can help keep your gut flora in check while avoiding unnecessary antibiotics that can prevent the decimation of beneficial bacteria that safeguard against overgrowth. Managing stress is also vital, as chronic stress can weaken your immune system and make your gut more susceptible to imbalances, including Candida overgrowth.

In essence, tackling Candida overgrowth requires a comprehensive approach that includes dietary modifications, probiotic support, and lifestyle changes. By understanding and addressing the root causes and contributing factors, you can restore and maintain a healthy balance in your gut, keeping Candida and other opportunistic microbes in check. This alleviates the troubling symptoms associated with overgrowth and enhances your overall health and well-being, allowing you to live a more balanced, energetic life, free from the disruptive influence of Candida.

2.5 UNDERSTANDING FOOD INTOLERANCES AND ALLERGIES

Let's unravel the often-confusing world of food intolerances and allergies, which, believe it or not, are as distinct from each other as apples and oranges. Understanding these differences is crucial for managing your diet and keeping your gut happy and healthy. Food intolerances often involve the digestive system's inability to handle certain foods. On the other hand, allergies are your immune system's overreaction to a food it mistakenly believes is harmful.

Food intolerances can vary widely, but they generally don't involve the immune system. Common culprits include lactose, found in dairy products, and gluten, found in wheat, rye, and barley. If your body struggles to digest these, it might respond with symptoms such as bloating, gas, or diarrhea. Now, allergies are a different beast. They can cause more severe reactions, including hives, swelling, difficulty breathing, and, in extreme cases, anaphylaxis—a potentially life-threatening reaction. These symptoms can kick in fast and furious, often within minutes of exposure to the offending food.

Identifying what's causing your symptoms can sometimes feel like trying to solve a mystery without all the clues. However, tools such as elimination diets can be incredibly revealing. This approach involves removing suspected foods from your diet for a period, then gradually reintroducing them while noting any symptoms. It's like conducting your own science experiment to see how your body reacts to different foods.

Another method is food challenges, often performed under medical supervision, where you consume the food in question in a controlled setting to monitor any adverse reactions.

Living with food intolerances requires a strategy that blends vigilance with flexibility. It's about making educated choices without feeling like you're missing out. Start by becoming a label-reading ninja, knowing precisely what's in your foods. Cooking from scratch can be a game-changer, giving you complete control over what goes into your meals. And let's remember the power of alternatives. Lactose-free dairy, gluten-free grains, and nut-free butter can be lifesavers, allowing you to enjoy your meals without the unpleasant aftermath.

Finding a balance that works for your lifestyle and body is essential in navigating these waters. Each person's reaction to food can be as unique as their fingerprint, and what works for one might not work for another. It's about tuning in to your body's signals and adjusting accordingly. By embracing this approach, you manage your symptoms more effectively and enhance your overall quality of life, ensuring that your diet supports your health without letting food intolerances dictate your choices.

In wrapping up this exploration of food intolerances and allergies, remember that the key is understanding the nuances of your body's responses and managing them proactively. This isn't just about avoiding discomfort. It's about empowering yourself to make choices that enhance your health and well-being. By clarifying what triggers your symptoms and how to manage them, you set the stage for more informed, health- conscious decisions that keep your gut feeling good and your body functioning well.

As we close this chapter, we've armed ourselves with essential insights into common gut issues and how to tackle them head-on. From unraveling the complexities of IBS and SIBO to addressing leaky gut and Candida overgrowth, and finally, differentiating and managing food intolerances and allergies, our journey through these topics isn't just about symptom management—it's about fostering a deeper understanding of our body's unique needs and responses. This knowledge is not merely functional, it's transformative, offering us the tools to improve our digestive health and enhance our overall quality of life.

As we turn the page, let's carry forward this empowering knowledge, ready to dive deeper into the dietary strategies that can help us maintain a healthy and vibrant gut. We will explore the roles of various diets and foods in nurturing our digestive health and ensuring our gut health is excellent and plentiful!

CHAPTER THREE
DIET'S ROLE IN GUT HEALTH

A h, diet. That ever-persistent buzzword that can either make us feel like a million bucks or the exact opposite, depending on the day, right? But let's not just talk about diet in the sense of dropping a few pounds or fitting into the skinny jeans tucked away in the back of your closet. No, let's talk about how your diet profoundly shapes the bustling metropolis that is your gut microbiome. Imagine each meal as a direct deposit into your gut's bank account, where the right kind of nutrients can make your gut flora thrive like a booming economy.

3.1 FOODS THAT HEAL YOUR GUT

Nourishing the Microbiome

First things first: the residents of your gut city, those trillions of bacteria, need the right food to flourish. We're talking about whole foods rich in fiber, prebiotics, and probiotics. Think of fiber as the city's infrastructure—roads and bridges—that keeps everything moving smoothly. Foods like bananas, oats, and flaxseeds keep you regular and help create a supportive environment for beneficial bacteria to thrive.

On the other hand, prebiotics are like the premium fuel for these good bacteria. They're found in foods like garlic, onions, and asparagus, feeding the good microbes and helping them multiply. Probiotics, found in yogurt and sauerkraut, add more beneficial bacteria to the mix, enhancing the diversity and resilience of your gut ecosystem. It's like throwing a block party where the whole neighborhood comes out, gets along famously, and cleans up the streets while they're at it.

Anti-inflammatory Foods

Now, onto the fire department of your gut city—anti-inflammatory foods. Inflammation can be a silent alarm, indicating trouble throughout the body, and often starts in the gut. To quiet this alarm, foods rich in omega-3 fatty acids like salmon, chia seeds, and walnuts are your go-to firefighters.

They work by reducing the inflammatory responses in your body, ensuring that chronic inflammation doesn't throw a wrench in your gut's daily operations. It's like having a state-of-the-art fire suppression system that keeps minor flare-ups from becoming full-blown infernos.

Bone Broth Benefits

Speaking of restoration, let's simmer down with some bone broth, shall we? This liquid gold is rich in collagen, like the cement that repairs roads and buildings in your gut city. Collagen helps heal and strengthen the gut lining, preventing unwanted substances from leaking into your bloodstream—yes, we're talking about leaky gut syndrome here. Sipping on bone broth can be as soothing to your gut as a spa day is for you after a long, stressful week.

Diversity is Key

Lastly, diversity would be its strength if your gut were a garden. Just as a well-tended garden has a mix of flowers, fruits, and vegetables, a healthy gut needs a variety of foods. This diversity encourages a robust microbiome, which can withstand and recover from challenges more effectively. Including a wide range of fruits, vegetables, whole grains, and proteins in your diet provides different nutrients that various bacteria in your gut need to perform their best. It's like hosting an international food festival in your gut—everyone finds something they love, and the whole system benefits from the variety.

Reflection Section: Your Gut's Dietary Palette

Let's take a moment to reflect on this array of gut-nourishing foods. How diverse is your current diet? Are you the type to stick to the same meals week in and week out, or are you constantly spicing things up with new recipes and ingredients? Consider jotting down what you eat over a week and then looking for patterns. Are you leaning heavily on processed foods? Is there a rainbow of fruits and vegetables on your plate, or is it more monochrome? This little audit isn't about feeling guilty or patting yourself on the back. It's about seeing where there might be room for more variety and balance, ensuring your gut microbiome is as vibrant and diverse as possible.

Incorporating these gut-healthy foods into your diet isn't just about dodging digestive discomfort or keeping your microbiome merry. It's a foundational strategy for boosting overall health and vitality. By choosing foods that nourish your gut, reduce inflammation, and maintain the integrity of your gut lining, you're not just eating— you're curating a lifestyle that supports your body's complex systems in performing their best. And the best part? This approach to eating doesn't require a complete overhaul of your diet. It's about making mindful choices that profoundly impact your health and well-being, one meal at a time. So, here's to delicious, diverse, and gut- nourishing foods that satisfy your taste buds and support your health from the inside out. Cheers to that, right?

3.2 THE TRUTH ABOUT FIBER AND GUT HEALTH

Diving deeper into gut health, we encounter fiber, a key player in our digestive wellness. It is often lauded for its role in digestion, yet sometimes it is not fully appreciated for its variety and impact on our gut ecosystem. Fiber is categorized into two primary types: insoluble and soluble, each serving an indispensable role in our digestive process. It transforms into a gel-like substance, enabling it to bind with fatty acids and slow down stomach emptying, keeping you satiated longer and helping stabilize blood sugar levels. Soluble fiber sources such as oats, apples, carrots, and beans offer a delicious array for those aiming to maintain a smooth digestive flow.

Conversely, insoluble fiber, which does not dissolve in water, adds bulk to your stool, functioning like a sweeping brush that moves through your digestive system, preventing constipation and ensuring regular bowel movements. Sources of insoluble fiber include whole grains, nuts, potatoes, and green leafy vegetables, providing a robust selection for a healthy diet. Together, these fiber types form a synergistic pair that supports digestion and plays a significant role in heart health and weight management, acting like an efficient cleaning service for your body's internal operations.

Among the fiber family stars is prebiotic fiber, a special kind of soluble fiber critical for gut health because it nurtures the growth of beneficial gut bacteria.

Prebiotic fibers are the preferred nutrition for gut microbes. They are not digested but journey to your lower digestive tract, serving as a feast for beneficial bacteria and fostering their growth and activity. High prebiotic fiber foods such as chicory root, garlic, onions, and leeks effectively host a banquet for your gut's friendly bacteria, bolstering everything from immune function to mood. Investing in your microbiome through these foods yields widespread health benefits.

Addressing practical considerations—how much fiber is optimal in your diet? The current recommendations advise about 25 to 30 grams of fiber daily from foods, not supplements, a goal many fail to achieve. To illustrate, an apple with its skin provides roughly 4.4 grams of fiber, while a cup of cooked lentils offers about 15.6 grams.

Consider this a fiscal plan for your gut health, allocating sufficient resources to flourish without excess. To integrate fiber into your diet effortlessly, add fiber-rich foods into one meal daily, like adding berries to your breakfast or choosing carrot sticks over chips for lunch. Gradually, allow your body to adjust, increasing your intake to reach your daily fiber goal. Modifying the pace at which you increase your fiber intake is essential. A sudden shift from a low-fiber to a high-fiber diet can shock your system, leading to bloating, gas, and discomfort, akin to an abrupt, intense workout for a sedentary individual. Your digestive system requires time to adapt to the added volume. To avoid these issues, gradually increase your fiber intake and drink ample water, facilitating smoother fiber passage through your system and mitigating discomfort and complications. This approach is a gentle, considerate prompt to your digestive system, signaling beneficial changes are on the horizon, undertaken together.

Mastering your dietary fiber intake transcends mere digestive aid —it's an essential element of your overarching health strategy, affecting everything from gut bacteria balance to chronic disease risk. Understanding fiber types and their unique benefits and strategically increasing your fiber intake while monitoring your body's reaction pave the way for a healthier, more content gut. Adopting a balanced, mindful diet as the foundation of digestive health and overall well-being signifies a simple yet profound commitment to your health journey. Hence, when contemplating your next meal or snack, view fiber as your dietary companion, steadfast in supporting your well-being with every bite. That fabulous friend to our gut health is often celebrated for its digestive benefits but is sometimes misunderstood for its diversity and impact on our gut ecosystem. Fiber comes in two main types: soluble and insoluble, each playing a unique and crucial role in our digestive ballet. Imagine soluble fiber as a sponge, absorbing water as it travels through your digestive tract. This transformation into a gel-like substance allows it to bind with fatty acids and prolong stomach emptying, which means it helps you feel full longer and can help regulate blood sugar. Foods rich in soluble fiber include apples, oats, carrots, and beans—a veritable feast for those looking to keep things smooth and steady.

Conversely, insoluble fiber is the roughage type that doesn't dissolve in water and adds bulk to your stool. This type of fiber acts like a broom, sweeping through your digestive tract and keeping things moving along, which helps prevent constipation and keeps your bowel movements regular. Whole grains, nuts, potatoes, and green leafy vegetables are go-to sources for this type of fiber. Together, these two types of fiber create a dynamic duo that supports digestion and contributes to heart health and weight management. It's like having a well-rounded cleaning crew that tidies up and ensures all systems run efficiently and smoothly.

Let's move on to the powerhouse of the fiber family: prebiotic fiber. This particular type of soluble fiber plays a crucial role in gut health by fostering the growth of beneficial bacteria in your gut. Think of prebiotic fibers as the ultimate health food for your gut microbes. They don't get digested but head straight to your lower digestive tract, which acts as a feast for your good bacteria, encouraging them to multiply and thrive. Foods high in prebiotic fiber include chicory root, garlic, onions, and leeks. By integrating these foods into your diet, you're throwing a dinner party for your gut's beneficial bacteria, helping to improve everything from your immune function to your mood. It's an investment in your microbiome that pays off in comprehensive health dividends.

Navigating the fibrous waters of your diet doesn't just aid your digestion—it's a critical component of your overall health strategy, influencing everything from your gut bacteria to your likelihood of chronic disease. Understanding the types of fiber and their unique benefits, and strategically increasing your fiber intake while observing your body's response, set the stage for a healthier, happier gut. It's a straightforward yet impactful approach to wellness that champions a balanced, thoughtful diet as the cornerstone of digestive health and holistic well-being. So, as you ponder your next meal or snack, think of fiber as your dietary ally, ready to support your health journey with every bite.

3.3 NAVIGATING THE WORLD OF FERMENTED FOODS

Let's get a little bubbly—not with champagne, but with something just as celebratory for your gut: fermented foods. Before you wrinkle your nose at the thought of bacteria and yeast partying in your food, consider these microbe-rich foods like a live concert for your gut, where beneficial bacteria are the stars. You get to enjoy the health benefits. Fermentation isn't just a modern dietary fad. It's a time-honored tradition that has been jazzing up diets around the globe for centuries. This process, essentially, is all about transformation. It starts with microorganisms, such as bacteria or yeast, breaking down sugars and starches in food, turning them into acids, gases, or alcohol. Not only does this add a zing to the flavors, but it also preserves the food and enhances its nutritional profile.

Fermented foods are probiotic powerhouses. These include everyday favorites like yogurt and kefir, as well as the tangy duo of sauerkraut and kimchi. Each food brings a unique blend of bacteria to help balance your gut flora, boosting digestion and overall health. Yogurt, for instance, is filled with lactobacilli, a friendly bacterium that can ease lactose digestion and rebalance gut flora after a round of antibiotics. Kefir, a fermented milk drink, offers a broader array of bacteria and yeasts, making it a potent probiotic.

Then there's sauerkraut and kimchi, both made from fermented cabbage, which not only supports gut health but is also loaded with vitamins C and K, plus iron—all of which are great for your overall well-being.

Incorporating these fermented delights into your diet can seem daunting if you're new to the world of beneficial bacteria. The key is to start small. Begin by introducing small servings of fermented foods into your meals. Think of a spoonful of sauerkraut on your sausage, a dollop of yogurt on your morning granola, or a shot glass of kefir as a quick snack. As your taste buds and digestive system get accustomed to these new flavors and sensations, gradually increase your portions. It's like acclimating to a hot bath — one toe at a time. This method helps avoid potential discomfort, such as bloating or gas if your body isn't used to digesting these probiotic-rich foods.

Now, if you're feeling adventurous and love a good DIY project, why not try fermenting at home? It's easier than you think, and you don't need a lab or special equipment to get started. A simple, fun entry into the world of fermentation is making your own sauerkraut. All you need is cabbage, salt, and a jar. The process involves thinly slicing the cabbage, mixing it with salt, and then packing it tightly in a jar. The salt draws out the water from the cabbage, creating a brine that submerges the cabbage. Natural fermentation occurs over several days to a few weeks, and voila— you've made your probiotic masterpiece! Just remember, when fermenting at home, cleanliness is crucial. Ensure all your tools and containers are well-sanitized to avoid unwanted bacterial growth.

Embracing fermented foods is like turning your meals into a daily celebration of flavors and cultures. These foods not only promise a delightful tang and zest to your dishes but also profoundly benefit your digestive health, packing every bite with beneficial bacteria that help keep your gut in top form. So why not let these microbial marvels jazz up your eating routine? Whether through a store-bought sampler of fermented goods or diving into home fermentation, each step you take enriches your diet, making each meal not just food but a nourishment for your body and your microbes.

3.4 THE ANTI-INFLAMMATORY DIET FOR GUT HEALTH

When it comes to soothing your gut and keeping the rest of your body humming without the fiery sparks of inflammation, think of your diet as an excellent, calm, collected friend who knows how to ease a heated situation. Did you know that some foods you eat can fan the flames of inflammation in your body? It's like throwing gasoline on a fire, except the fire is in your gut, and the gas is some of your favorite comfort foods. Conversely, the right foods can be like a soothing balm, dousing the flames and restoring peace. This is where the anti-inflammatory diet steps into the limelight, not just as a diet but as a lifestyle choice that helps manage inflammation, potentially easing chronic pain and preventing various health issues.

So, what fuels this inflammation? Often, it's a diet laden with overly processed foods, excessive sugars, and certain unsavory oils that tip the balance toward inflammation. These foods can trigger a cascade of reactions, leading to chronic inflammation that just doesn't quit. It's like leaving a slow burner under a pot - eventually, things will boil over. To counter this, an anti-inflammatory diet focuses on just the opposite foods.

Imagine your plate loaded with vibrant fruits and vegetables, lean proteins, and healthy fats, all known to combat inflammation. It's not just about cutting out the bad stuff. It's about packing all the good stuff your body loves.

Fruits and vegetables are stars in this dietary lineup because they're high in natural antioxidants and polyphenols—protective compounds that help reduce inflammation. Whether it's the deep blues of blueberries, the vibrant oranges of sweet potatoes, or the lush greens of spinach, these foods are not just color splashes on your plate. They're potent allies in your fight against inflammation. Lean proteins like chicken, turkey, and fish are also crucial. They provide the necessary building blocks for your body without the extra fats contributing to inflammation. And let's not forget about the healthy fats, particularly those famed omega-3 fatty acids found in fish like salmon and in flaxseeds, celebrated for their anti-inflammatory properties.

Switching gears to what you should avoid can make just as much of an impact. Processed foods and sugars are the usual suspects, lurking in the shadows of your snack drawer, ready to stir up trouble. These foods are low in nutritional value and high in ingredients that trigger inflammation. Similarly, oils like soybean and corn, high in omega-6 fatty acids, can tip your body's balance toward inflammation if consumed in excess. It's all about striking the right balance between omega-6s and omega-3s. The goal is to avoid these inflammation culprits and replace them with healthier alternatives contributing to your well-being. For example, swapping out vegetable oils for something more stable and less inflammatory, like olive or avocado, can be a simple yet effective change.

Now, let's talk about meal planning because, let's face it, the best intentions can only fall flat without a plan. Planning meals around an anti-inflammatory diet doesn't have to be a chore or mean giving up delicious foods. It's about making smarter choices that align with your health goals. Start by building your meals around a core of anti- inflammatory foods. It could be a salmon fillet with steamed broccoli and quinoa or a vibrant salad with mixed greens, colorful veggies, nuts, and olive oil dressing. The key is to consider each meal an opportunity to nourish and protect your body rather than just filling up. And yes, you can still have desserts and treats —opt for those made with less sugar and healthier ingredients. Dark chocolate, rich in antioxidants, can be a great option in moderation.

Embracing an anti-inflammatory diet is like signing a peace treaty with your body. It's a commitment to reducing the internal skirmishes that inflammation can cause, leading to a healthier, more vibrant you. By choosing foods that heal rather than harm, you're taking a proactive step toward managing inflammation and all its complications. So next time you plot your meals, think of each ingredient as a peacekeeper, and you'll be well on your way to a calmer, more nourished body.

3.5 FOODS TO AVOID FOR OPTIMAL GUT HEALTH

When it comes to maintaining a happy gut, sometimes what you don't eat is just as important as what you do eat. Think of your gut as a VIP party—while you want to invite all the nutrients that make your gut thrive, there are also a few uninvited guests that you should probably keep off the guest list. Processed foods, for instance, are like those party crashers who bring nothing to the table but trouble. Combined with high sugar content and a cocktail of artificial additives, these foods can turn your gut microbiome into a scene of microbial mayhem. The simple sugars and refined flours in processed foods are gobbled up quickly by harmful bacteria, allowing them to increase, pushing out the beneficial bacteria. It's like feeding the bullies who take over the playground, leaving little room for the good kids.

Let's talk about two popular beverages that might do more harm than good: alcohol and caffeine. Now, enjoying a glass of wine or a morning coffee in moderation isn't a crime, but tipping the scales towards excessive consumption can ruffle some feathers in your gut lining. Alcohol, particularly in larger quantities, can irritate your gut wall, leading to inflammation and even contributing to the leakage of harmful bacteria into your bloodstream. It's akin to throwing a wild party in your gut where things get out of hand, resulting in calls to the police—or, in this case, your immune system.

Conversely, caffeine can be like that friend who talks a mile a minute, ramping up your stress hormones, which, in turn, can mess with your digestion and microbial balance. Sugar deserves special mention for its role in dysbiosis, a microbial imbalance in your gut. High sugar intake can lead to an overgrowth of harmful bacteria and yeast, like weeds overtaking a garden. These microorganisms thrive on sugar, and when they multiply, they can edge out the beneficial bacteria, disrupting your gut's harmony. It's like sugar fertilizes the weeds, allowing them to spread out of control, choking the beautiful flowers and plants you want to thrive.

While it's important to recognize these general gut health offenders, it's equally crucial to tune into your body's responses. Each person's gut reacts differently to various foods, so identifying your triggers is critical. This process involves listening to your body and noting how it responds to different foods. Think of it like being a detective in your health mystery—keeping a food diary, noting symptoms, and maybe even working with a nutritionist or healthcare provider to analyze the clues. This proactive approach allows you to tailor your diet to support your gut health, ensuring your gut microbiome can thrive in its unique ecosystem.

By steering clear of processed foods, moderating your intake of alcohol and caffeine, cutting down on sugars, and pinpointing your personal food triggers, you can help maintain a balanced and healthy gut. It's about making conscious choices that support your microbial community, ensuring that your gut remains a welcoming place for beneficial bacteria and not a free-for-all that leads to discomfort and disease.

As we wrap up this chapter on the pivotal role of diet in gut health, we've journeyed through the best foods to include and those to avoid for maintaining a vibrant, healthy gut. From the powerhouses of fiber and anti-inflammatory foods to the cultured world of fermented delights and mindful avoidance of gut disruptors, your diet shapes your gut health and, by extension, your overall well-being. As you continue to navigate your dietary choices, remember that each meal is an opportunity to support your gut and your entire body's health.

Looking ahead, we'll explore how lifestyle factors beyond diet, including stress management and sleep, play a crucial role in gut health. It's not just about what you eat but also how you live. So, stay tuned as we continue to unravel the complex, fascinating world of gut health, ensuring you're equipped to lead a healthier, happier life.

CHAPTER FOUR

SUPPLEMENTS FOR GUT HEALTH

A h, the world of supplements! It's like navigating a bustling bazaar in a far-flung land. Every stall and vendor promises miracles in a bottle—or, in this case, a pill. But before you throw your money at the most colorful label or the sales pitch that tugs at your heartstrings, let's talk seriously about gut health supplements.

4.1 THE ESSENTIAL GUIDE TO PROBIOTIC SUPPLEMENTS

Choosing the Right Probiotic

Diving into the sea of probiotic supplements without a compass can be like trying to find a needle in a haystack. It's a delicious, beneficial, bacteria-filled haystack, but a haystack, nonetheless. The first thing you should look for in a probiotic supplement is the specific strains of bacteria it contains. Not all bacteria are created equal. Different strains have different powers. For instance, Lactobacillus acidophilus is excellent for digestion and warding off vaginal infections, while Bifidobacterium bifidum can help strengthen your immune system.

Next, let's talk numbers—CFUs or colony-forming units, which tell you how many bacteria in the probiotics are expected to set up camp in your gut. Generally, a higher CFU count (think billions) might imply more potency, but only if those little critters are alive through the expiration date. Yep, these bacteria need to be alive to set up shop in your gut and get to work! Always check the label for viability, ensuring these organisms will be alive and kicking when it's time for them to do their job.

Health Benefits

Probiotics are like the superheroes of your gut, each with unique powers that contribute to your health's storyline. Regularly taking probiotic supplements can lead to plot twists, from improved digestion and reduced symptoms of irritable bowel syndrome to enhanced immune function. Think of them as your health allies, tiny as they are, battling the bad guys and keeping the peace in the bustling city of your gut.

But the benefits aren't just about fighting villains and maintaining the peace. For women, this can mean keeping things like yeast infections and urinary tract infections at bay, thanks to a well-balanced vaginal flora. Plus, for those who often feel like their stomach is in knots or who face the wrath of bloating, probiotics can help calm the storms, ensuring smoother sailing and better digestive health.

Supplements vs. Food Sources

Should you get these bacterial benefits from a pill or a plate? While fermented foods like yogurt, kefir, and sauerkraut are natural probiotic champions, supplements offer a more concentrated dose of specific beneficial bacteria. It is like choosing between a multivitamin and eating several pounds of fruits and vegetables. Sometimes, you need that extra punch that only a supplement can provide.

However, supplements aren't without their cons. They can be pricey, and navigating the myriad options can be overwhelming. Plus, relying solely on supplements can lead you to miss out on the other nutritional benefits that come from probiotic-rich foods, like the fiber in sauerkraut or the protein in yogurt. Ideally, a combo meal—part food, part supplement—is a balanced approach to ensuring your gut gets what it needs.

Safety and Side Effects

While probiotics are generally safe because they're composed of bacteria already present in a regular digestive system, they can cause some side effects, especially when you first start taking them. These can include gas, bloating, or discomfort, which is your digestive system's way of saying, "Whoa, who are all these new folks?" These effects are mild and temporary for most people as the body adjusts.

However, for those with compromised immune systems or existing health conditions, probiotics can sometimes cause more severe side effects. Always talk to your healthcare provider before starting a new supplement, especially if you have health concerns.

Reflective Section: Your Probiotic Needs

Let's pause for a gut check—literally. Reflect on what your digestive system needs. Are you frequently battling stomach upsets? Do you feel like your immune system could use a boost? Or maybe you're just aiming for overall well-being? Understanding your body's needs can help you more easily navigate the bustling market of probiotics.

Consider keeping a symptom diary, jotting down your digestive highs and lows, and discussing these with a healthcare provider who can help guide your probiotic choices effectively.

In the grand bazaar of supplements, armed with the proper knowledge, you can make choices that suit your gut's needs and support your overall health journey. As we explore other supplements in the following sections, remember that each piece of the puzzle is crucial to creating a complete picture of health, one little pill—or food choice—at a time.

4.2 PREBIOTICS: THE FUEL FOR YOUR GUT FLORA

Turning our attention to prebiotics, we see that these foundational elements of gut health often fly under the radar compared to their counterparts, probiotics. Picture prebiotics as the essential nourishment that cultivates a thriving community of beneficial gut bacteria. These indigestible fibers journey through the digestive tract largely unaltered, reaching the colon and serving as a vital food source for the friendly bacteria living there.

Understanding prebiotics begins with recognizing their source: your diet. Unlike probiotics, which are living organisms, prebiotics are found in types of carbohydrates (primarily fibers) that humans cannot digest. The primary role of these nutrients is to stimulate the growth and activity of advantageous bacteria in the gut. This can lead to various benefits for overall health, including enhancing digestion, improving calcium absorption, and lowering the risk of cardiovascular disease. Essentially, without prebiotics, your probiotics would be like gardeners without seeds. They'd have little to work with.

Look at your kitchen if you're wondering where to get these marvelous meal-makers. Prebiotics are abundant in many common foods, particularly in the fiber-rich ones.

Garlic and onions add flavor to nearly any dish and include inulin and oligofructose, which are superstar prebiotics. Slightly green bananas are great for a prebiotic boost with their resistant starch. Whole grains like barley and oats are loaded with beta-glucan, a prebiotic fiber that helps your gut bacteria thrive and improves cholesterol levels and heart health. Integrating these foods into your diet isn't just about keeping your gut happy. It's about creating a cascade of health benefits that ripple throughout your body.

It would be best to have more prebiotics in your diet, and that's where supplements step in. Supplementing with prebiotics offers a direct, controlled way to boost your gut flora. When choosing a prebiotic supplement, look for products that specify the type of fibers or compounds they contain, such as inulin, FOS (fructooligosaccharides), or GOS (galactooligosaccharides). Quality matters because you want a product that effectively feeds your good bacteria without contributing to any digestive discomfort, which can sometimes occur if you dive too deep, too fast into the world of fiber.

The real magic happens when prebiotics and probiotics are combined. This dynamic duo works synergistically to enhance your gut health more effectively than either would alone. This combination, often called synbiotics, ensures that the probiotics have the necessary nutrients to thrive and benefit your gut. Whether you get these through your diet or supplements, providing a balance of prebiotics and probiotics can help you maintain an optimal environment for gut health, paving the way to improved well-being. So, as you consider your dietary choices or the supplements aisle, think of prebiotics as the key to unlocking the full potential of your gut bacteria. By ensuring these microscopic chefs have all they need to cook up a storm of health benefits, you're setting the stage for a healthier, more vibrant you. Remember, every bite or supplement you take can be a step towards a happier gut, a healthier body, and perhaps even a brighter mood.

4.3 SUPPLEMENTS FOR COMBATING LEAKY GUT

Consider supplements as your handy tool kit when giving your gut a bit of TLC, especially if you're dealing with the notorious leaky gut. Imagine your gut lining as a garden hose - water flows freely and directly to where it's needed when it's in top shape. But water leaks when holes are in the hose, causing a mess. A leaky gut is similar, letting substances into your bloodstream that shouldn't be there, which can lead to a cascade of health issues. But fear not because a whole arsenal of supplements is designed to patch up your gut lining and restore order in your digestive tract.

Let's start with L-glutamine, an amino acid, like the handyman of gut repair. This isn't just any supplement. It's a frontline warrior in the battle against gut permeability. L- glutamine fuels the cells that line your intestines, helping repair and regenerate them. It's like providing bricks and mortar to a wall that needs rebuilding. Regularly adding L- glutamine to your diet can help strengthen the barrier of your intestines, making it harder for unwanted substances to pass through. Think of it as fortifying the gates of your castle, keeping the marauders out and the peace in. L- glutamine is your go-to whether you're recovering from intense exercise, dealing with the stress that hits your gut hard, or just looking to maintain a strong and healthy digestive system.

Let's talk about Omega-3 fatty acids, known for their anti-inflammatory prowess. These aren't just good for your heart, they're like the peacekeepers of your body, calming inflammation and helping to maintain the integrity of your gut lining. In fish oil, flaxseeds, and chia seeds, Omega-3s help soothe the gut by reducing inflammation that can exacerbate leaky gut. Integrating Omega-3 supplements into your regimen is like sending in a specialized clean-up crew after a riot—restoring order and ensuring everything runs smoothly.

Remember herbal allies like slippery elm, marshmallow root, and licorice root. These aren't just old wives' tales. Each of these herbs has properties that help soothe the gut lining and promote healing. Slippery elm and marshmallow root provide a mucilage or gel-like substance that coats the gut lining, acting as a balm for irritated or inflamed tissues. It's similar to applying a soothing lotion to a sunburn. They're the herbal equivalent of a gentle hug for your insides, calming inflammation and protecting against further irritation. Licorice root, which should be used in its deglycyrrhizinated form to avoid side effects, has anti-inflammatory and immune-boosting properties, making it a triple benefit to gut health.

Last but certainly not least, let's dive into collagen peptides. These small proteins are derived from collagen, a vital component of the gut lining. Think of collagen peptides as the protein shake for your gut cells. They provide the building blocks for repairing and maintaining a healthy intestinal barrier. Regularly including collagen peptides in your diet can help your gut lining stay as strong and flexible as a brand-new yoga mat, ready to bend without breaking. Whether added to your morning smoothie or nightly tea, collagen peptides are an easy and effective way to support your gut health.

Each supplement offers a unique blend of benefits tailored to reinforce your gut lining and ensure it functions at its best. By choosing the right combination of supplements, you're not just patching holes but building a more robust, healthier digestive system that can stand up to whatever life throws. So, as you consider your supplement strategy, think of it as equipping your gut with the best tools for the job—tools ready to repair, rejuvenate, and revitalize your digestive health.

4.4 VITAMINS AND MINERALS CRITICAL FOR DIGESTIVE HEALTH

Let's turn our attention to the unsung heroes of our digestive saga —the vitamins and minerals that play pivotal roles yet often don't get the spotlight they deserve.

Vitamin D and Gut Health

First up is Vitamin D, famously known as the "sunshine vitamin," but its role extends well beyond keeping our bones healthy. Recent spotlights have been shining on its relationship with gut health, and let me tell you, it's quite the dynamic duo. Vitamin D receptors are found throughout the gut, playing a crucial role in shaping the microbial community. Vitamin D holds a managerial position, overseeing various aspects of gut function, from immune response modulation to maintaining the gut barrier.

Low Vitamin D levels have been linked with an increased risk of inflammatory bowel diseases like Crohn's and ulcerative colitis and a more general increase in gut inflammation. It's like when the manager is out of the office—the processes don't run as smoothly, and things can go awry. Ensuring you have enough Vitamin D through diet, supplementation, or sun exposure helps keep the gut's immune responses and barrier functions in check.

Magnesium for Digestion

Next, let's talk about Magnesium. This mineral is somewhat of a multitasker in your body, involved in over 300 biochemical reactions—think of it as the utility player on your favorite sports team. Magnesium's role is crucial yet often overlooked when it comes to digestion. It helps relax the muscles in your digestive tract, including the intestines, which allows food movement along the gut. This process, known as peristalsis, is essential for regular bowel movements.

Magnesium also acts as a natural antacid. Neutralizing stomach acid helps create a friendlier environment where food can be properly broken down. For those who occasionally struggle with constipation, Magnesium might be the gentle nudge your system needs. It draws water into the intestines, softening the stool and making it easier to pass. A magnesium-rich diet is like having a sound traffic management system; it keeps things moving smoothly along the highway, which is your digestive tract.

Zinc's Healing Properties

Now, let's sprinkle some Zinc into the mix. Zinc is like the repair technician of your body, especially when it comes to maintaining the gut lining. It significantly affects wound healing and immune function, directly to gut health. A robust gut barrier is essential to prevent pathogens and toxins from entering the bloodstream—a process we've touched on earlier called leaky gut syndrome.

Zinc's role in supporting the immune system also means it's vital for combating inflammation and infection in the gut. Think of Zinc as a superhero, swooping in to repair damage and fight off bad guys that might compromise your gut health. Ensuring you have enough Zinc in your diet, whether through food sources like meat, shellfish, legumes, or supplements, can help keep your gut lining strong and your immune responses sharp.

Iron Absorption and Gut Health

Lastly, let's delve into Iron and its complex relationship with gut health. Iron is critical in making hemoglobin, the protein in your blood that helps transport oxygen around your body. But here's the twist: Iron absorption heavily depends on your gut's health. An inflamed or unhealthy gut can severely hamper your body's ability to absorb Iron, leading to iron deficiency anemia, leaving you tired and weak.

Moreover, the type of Iron in your diet matters. Heme iron, found in animal products, is generally absorbed better than non-heme Iron from plant sources. However, vitamin C can boost the absorption of non-heme Iron, so pairing iron-rich plant foods with something like orange juice can be a great strategy. It's all about ensuring the stage is set for Iron to make its best appearance in the play of digestion, providing your body gets the oxygen it needs to keep all systems, including your gut, running smoothly.

As we wrap up this exploration of the vital roles vitamins and minerals play in your digestive health, remember that each nutrient is crucial in the intricate dance of digestion and overall health. Whether it's the immune-modulating actions of Vitamin D, the muscle-relaxing prowess of Magnesium, the reparative properties of Zinc, or the critical absorption of Iron, these nutrients ensure your digestive system performs at its best. By understanding their roles and ensuring you're getting enough of each, you're setting the stage for a healthier gut you.

Looking ahead, we'll continue to explore other crucial elements of gut health, including the impact of lifestyle factors such as stress and sleep. As with diet, these aspects play pivotal roles in maintaining a healthy gut and a vibrant, energetic life. Let's keep this momentum going as we move forward, equipped with knowledge and ready to take on the world, one healthy choice at a time.

CHAPTER FIVE

PRACTICAL LIFESTYLE CHANGES FOR GUT HEALTH

E nvision your gut as a vibrant city at peak traffic. Suddenly, a significant roadblock occurs—complete with blaring horns and the stress that brings traffic to a standstill. This scenario vividly illustrates what stress does to your digestive system. Much like a city operates optimally with a smooth traffic flow, your gut functions best when stress is effectively managed. This chapter delves into the intricate yet intimate connection between your brain and your gut. We'll introduce practical, transformative strategies to ensure the "traffic" within your internal ecosystem flows freely, avoiding the congestion caused by stress.

5.1 REDUCING STRESS FOR A HAPPIER GUT

Mind-Gut Connection: More Than Just a Feeling

Have you ever had butterflies in your stomach before a big presentation or felt a gut- wrenching sensation during stressful times? That's your brain and gut in deep conversation. Stress doesn't just mess with your mind. It physically alters your gut, including your gut bacteria, and ramps up inflammation. This is because your gut is sensitive to stress hormones, which can disrupt the delicate balance of your gut microbiome and make the intestinal lining more susceptible to inflammation.

Stress Management Techniques: Tools to Tame the Turmoil

Managing stress might not be as elusive as you think. Techniques like meditation, yoga, and deep breathing exercises aren't just new-age fluff; they are practical tools that can significantly lower stress levels and, consequently, soothe your gut.

Meditation: Think of meditation as your daily mental detox. Just as you might sip a green smoothie to cleanse your body, meditation clears your mind, reducing the clutter and chaos that stress thrives on. By focusing on your breath or a mantra, meditation helps calm the mind, which in turn calms the gut.

Yoga: More than just impressive poses, yoga is about creating balance in the body through strengthening and relaxing. The gentle stretches and poses in yoga help ease physical tension, alleviating stress-induced gut issues like bloating and pain. Plus, the emphasis on deep breathing helps to massage your abdominal organs, moving that gut traffic as smoothly as a well-directed symphony.

Deep Breathing Exercises: Have you ever noticed how your breathing becomes shallow and rapid when stressed? Deep breathing exercises are the antidote. You activate your body's natural relaxation response by consciously slowing down and deepening your breaths. This helps to slow down an overactive nervous system and reduce stress, giving your gut a break from the chaos.

Routine Importance: Crafting Calm in Your Daily Life

Establishing a calming routine isn't just about adding peace to your day. It's about subtracting stress from your life, which can have profound implications for your gut health. Start with simple integrations like a morning meditation, a midday yoga break, or evening deep breathing exercises. These practices help to set a calm tone for the day and can be incredibly effective at night to help wind down before sleep, reducing stress and improving gut health.

Creating a routine that incorporates these stress management techniques ensures that you're addressing stress at the moment and preventing it from accumulating. Think of it as regular maintenance for your internal city, keeping the streets clear, traffic moving without hitches, and controlling the gridlocks that can lead to chronic gut distress.

Long-Term Benefits: A Smooth Ride for Gut and Mind

The long-term benefits of reducing stress extend beyond occasional relief from bloating or indigestion. Chronic stress is a significant player in gut-related disorders like irritable bowel syndrome (IBS) and inflammatory bowel disease (IBD). By managing stress effectively, you're not just easing symptoms temporarily, you're potentially decreasing the risk of these disorders and promoting a more resilient digestive system. Moreover, the benefits of a calmer mind and a happier gut feed into each other. A less stressed mind promotes a healthier gut, which sends positive signals back to the brain, creating a virtuous cycle of health. It's a holistic approach that enhances your quality of life, proving that calm keeps your mind and gut running smoothly.

Interactive Element: Stress Management Action Plan

Why not create a Stress Management Action Plan to integrate these techniques into your life? Start by identifying the times of day when you feel most stressed. Assign a specific stress-reduction technique to each of these times. For instance, if mornings are hectic, try starting your day with five minutes of meditation. If afternoons are a struggle, incorporate a 15-minute yoga session during your lunch break. Customize this plan to fit your schedule and needs and watch your days and digestive health transform.

5.2 THE IMPORTANCE OF SLEEP FOR DIGESTIVE HEALTH

Imagine that your body is a sophisticated factory operating on a 24-hour schedule. At night, while you're nestled comfortably in your bed, the factory doesn't shut down.

Instead, it switches gears, moving from daytime activities to crucial overnight tasks, including restoring and rebalancing your gut microbiome. Quality sleep is like hitting the reset button for your digestive system, giving it the downtime it needs to repair, regenerate, and recalibrate. But when sleep evades you, it's not just your energy levels and mood that suffer. Your digestive health takes a hit, too.

The relationship between sleep and your gut is a two-way street. Not only does poor sleep disrupt your gut health, but an imbalanced gut can also lead to sleep disturbances. During sleep, your body regenerates cells and repairs tissues, including those in your gut. The microbiome also undergoes shifts in composition and activity, aligning with your body's circadian rhythms. Disrupt these rhythms—by skimping on sleep, for example—and you risk throwing these processes off balance. This can lead to an unhappy gut, manifesting as bloating, discomfort, and even increased food sensitivity. Essentially, missing out on sleep can create a kind of jet lag in your gut, with all the accompanying symptoms of digestive discomfort.

Now, let's talk about crafting the perfect environment for restorative sleep because setting the stage for good sleep is as important as the act itself. First, maintaining a regular sleep schedule helps synchronize your body's internal clock, or circadian rhythm, which governs your sleep-wake cycle and various functions in your gut. Going to bed and waking up at the same time every day—even on weekends—can significantly improve the quality of your sleep and, by extension, your gut health.

Creating a restful environment is critical. Your bedroom should be a sanctuary dedicated to rest. Invest in a good quality mattress and pillows to support your body and consider blackout curtains to shield against intrusive light. Keep the temperature cool, as a more relaxed room can help lower your body temperature, signaling to your body that it's time to sleep. Also, in the hour before bed, dim the lights and turn off electronic devices to help signal to your brain that it's time to wind down. These steps can make a big difference in your ability to fall asleep, ensuring your gut has a peaceful environment to carry out its nightly duties.

Sleep deprivation, unfortunately, is all too common, and its effects on gut health are more significant than many realize. Lack of sleep can increase the levels of stress hormones in your body, which inflame your gastrointestinal system and can disrupt the microbiome. This disruption can reduce the overall diversity of your gut bacteria, a critical factor in healthy digestion and immune function. Moreover, when you're sleep deprived, the body craves quick energy fixes—often in the form of high-sugar, high-fat foods—which can further throw your gut microbiome out of balance. It's a vicious cycle: poor sleep leads to poor dietary choices, negatively impacting gut health and potentially leading to more sleep issues.

Certain supplements can be beneficial in supporting both sleep and gut health. Magnesium, for instance, plays a dual role. It's crucial for muscle relaxation, which can aid in falling asleep, but it also has a calming effect on the gut, reducing spasms and discomfort. Melatonin, often called the sleep hormone, can regulate sleep patterns while also playing a protective role in the gut, reducing oxidative stress and inflammation. However, it's essential to approach these supplements with care, starting with low doses and, ideally, consulting with a healthcare provider to ensure they are a good fit for your specific health needs.

Incorporating these practices and considerations into your nightly routine can transform your sleep quality and digestive health. By prioritizing good sleep hygiene, you're not just resting your body. You're revitalizing your gut, ensuring it's ready to support you in all your waking hours.

5.3 EXERCISE AND GUT HEALTH: WHAT'S THE CONNECTION?

Lacing up those sneakers and hitting the gym, or even just walking around the block, might seem like it's all about burning calories or building muscle. But there's a hidden beneficiary to this physical activity—your gut. Regular exercise does more than sculpt your body. It also sculpts your gut microbiome, the community of microorganisms living inside you.

The perks of physical activity extend deep into your gut. Exercise increases the production of butyrate, a short-chain fatty acid that feeds the good bacteria in your gut. Think of butyrate as a gourmet meal for your microbes. It helps them grow and flourish, enhancing your gut health and boosting your immune system. Moreover, regular movement helps to stimulate the movement of your intestines, reducing the time food spends in your digestive system. This means less chance for fermentation, which can cause bloating and discomfort, and a healthier, happier gut environment.

Before sprinting to sign up for the next marathon, let's talk about what exercise can benefit your gut. Aerobic exercises, like swimming, cycling, or jogging, are fantastic because they increase your breathing and heart rate, enhancing the blood flow to your gut and muscles. This increased circulation helps to efficiently transport nutrients and oxygen throughout your body, aiding digestion and nutrient absorption. On the other hand, strength training, such as lifting weights or using resistance bands, might not immediately seem linked to gut health, but it plays a crucial role, too. It helps build muscle mass, improving insulin sensitivity, which can directly impact your gut by reducing inflammation.

The frequency and duration of exercise are also vital components. General guidelines suggest about 150 minutes of moderate aerobic activity and 75 minutes of vigorous activity per week, and muscle-strengthening exercises two or more days a week. However, it's not just about ticking boxes. It's about consistency and enjoyment. Integrating physical activity into your daily routine in a way that feels rewarding and doable is crucial. Whether it's a morning swim, a lunchtime walk, or an evening class at the gym, find what works for you and make it a regular part of your life.

However, it's essential to tailor your exercise regime to suit your health and fitness levels, especially to avoid gastrointestinal discomfort. For instance, high-intensity workouts can sometimes lead to digestive issues such as reflux, bloating, or diarrhea. This mainly happens when you dive in too fast without proper conditioning. Starting slowly and gradually increasing the intensity allows your body—and your gut—to adapt. It's also important to consider your hydration and nutrition before and after workouts. Ensuring you're well-hydrated and have eaten a suitable meal can significantly affect how your gut handles the exercise.

Remember, everybody is unique, and so is every gut. Attention to how your body responds to different exercise types can provide valuable clues about what works best for your digestive health. You may thrive on long bike rides but find that high-intensity interval training upsets your stomach. Or it's the other way around. Noticing these patterns isn't just about avoiding discomfort. It's about crafting a lifestyle that fosters physical and gut health. So, as you tie those laces or roll out that yoga mat, consider your physical activity's profound effects on your gut. With each step, pedal, or stretch, you're moving toward a fitter body and a more balanced, healthier gut.

5.4 HYDRATION: THE UNSUNG HERO OF GUT HEALTH

Water: The Essential Elixir for Digestive Well-being

Consider water a basic necessity and a vital component of your gut health. Amidst the buzz around superfoods and the latest dietary supplements, the fundamental role of water is too often understated.

Imagine your digestive system as complex machinery that relies on hydration to function smoothly. Without adequate water, breaking down food, absorbing nutrients, and maintaining a lubricated intestinal lining, the gut becomes compromised. This can slow digestion, leading to constipation and discomfort—an internal traffic jam where progress stalls and frustration builds. Essentially, water is critical to a seamless digestive journey, ensuring everything moves along as it should and keeping the environment in your gut optimized for health.

Hydration keeps things flowing and impact your gut's mucosal lining, which is the barrier protecting your internal tissues from your stomach's harsh, acidic environment. This lining needs to stay moist to protect and function properly. Recent studies have illuminated how hydration affects this mucosal barrier and, in turn, the balance of microbes in your gut. Proper hydration helps maintain the integrity of your gut's mucosal lining, supporting a healthy balance of gut bacteria, crucial for everything from digesting food to regulating your immune system. So, by staying hydrated, you're not just quenching your thirst—you're also nurturing a foundational aspect of your gut health, ensuring that your microbial partners are thriving in a well- maintained habitat.

So how much water should you drink? While the adage of eight glasses a day is a good baseline, the truth is that everyone's needs are different. Factors like your activity level, the climate you live in, your health status, and even what you eat (foods high in water content can contribute to your hydration) all play a role in determining your ideal water intake. A practical guideline to follow is the color of your urine—aim for light yellow. If it's clear, you might be overdoing it (yes, you can drink too much water). If it's dark, like the deep amber of a fine whiskey, it's time to hit the water bottle more often. Start your day with a glass of water and keep a bottle handy throughout the day, making it easier to sip regularly rather than chugging intermittently.

Being aware of the signs of dehydration can also help you stay on top of your hydration game before any severe red flags arise. Early signs include feeling thirsty, dry mouth, and decreased urine output. But let's not wait for your body to start screaming for moisture. More severe dehydration can lead to headache, dizziness, and extreme fatigue—signals that your body is running low on its essential fluid, and your gut health could be jeopardized. Chronic dehydration can lead to more persistent issues like constipation and an increased risk of urinary tract infections and kidney stones.

Incorporating more fluids into your day doesn't have to be a tedious task. If you find plain water monotonous, jazz it up with slices of lemon, cucumber, or fruit juice. Herbal teas are another excellent hydrator, often bringing their palette of health benefits, and they can be enjoyed hot or cold. Foods with high water content, such as watermelon, cucumber, and celery, also contribute to your hydration levels, offering a nutritious and hydrating snack option.

By understanding the critical role water plays in your overall health, specifically your digestive health, you can see hydration in a new light. It's not just about drinking enough water; it's about maintaining a fluid balance that supports every function of your body, from your brain to your gut. So next time you reach for a glass of water, remember, you're not just quenching thirst, you're facilitating a whole host of vital bodily functions, ensuring your gut is well-equipped to handle whatever comes its way with every sip.

5.5 MINDFUL EATING FOR OPTIMAL DIGESTION

Principles of Mindful Eating: More Than Just Chewing

Let's start with a truth bomb: how you eat can be just as crucial as what you eat. Mindful eating isn't about following an eating trend. It's about connecting more deeply with your eating experiences. It's a practice of being fully present during meals, paying attention to your food's flavors, textures, and sensations, and tuning into your body's hunger and fullness signals. This approach turns each meal into a moment of introspection and enjoyment rather than a mindless act of fueling up.

When you eat mindfully, you're nourishing your body and giving your digestive system the cue to perform at its best. You will likely chew your food more thoroughly by slowing down and savoring each bite. This not only makes digestion easier but also enhances nutrient absorption. After all, digestion begins in the mouth with the enzymatic action of saliva. The more you chew, the less work your stomach has to do, and the more smoothly the process goes. It's like prepping your food perfectly before tossing it into a well-oiled machine—everything runs smoother, and the results are better.

Mindful Eating Practices: Simple Steps to Savor

Implementing mindful eating can seem daunting, but it's all about starting small. One practical strategy is to eliminate distractions during meals. This means turning off the TV, putting away your phone, and focusing on your meal. It's about making your dining table a no-scroll zone. Try it at your next meal. You might be surprised by how much more you notice and enjoy your food.

Another essential practice is to slow down your eating pace. Set down your utensils between bites, chew thoroughly, and taste your food. This helps digestion and gives your brain time to catch up with your stomach. It takes about 20 minutes for your brain to receive signals of fullness from your stomach, so taking your time can prevent overeating and the discomfort that often follows.

You can also use mealtime as an opportunity to engage your senses fully. Notice the color, smell, and texture of your food. How does it feel in your mouth? How does its flavor change as you chew? Engaging your senses enhances your dining experience and deepens your connection to your food and its origins, which can be incredibly satisfying on more than just a culinary level.

Impact on Gut Health: A Calm Approach to Better Digestion

The benefits of mindful eating extend beyond the immediate pleasures of a good meal. By reducing your eating speed and increasing your awareness of hunger and fullness cues, you're less likely to engage in stress-related eating behaviors that can upset your digestive system. Stress eating often leads to consuming too much too quickly, not chewing properly, and choosing less nutritious comfort foods—all of which can wreak havoc on your gut.

Mindful eating practices cultivate a healthier relationship with food, which can lead to better choices and improved long-term digestive health. When you're more in tune with your body's needs, you're more likely to reach for what nourishes you rather than merely satisfies a momentary craving. This shift can reduce episodes of indigestion, bloating, and irregularity, as your gut isn't subjected to the rollercoaster of reactive eating habits.

Integrating Mindfulness into Meals: Making Every Bite Count

To effectively weave mindfulness into your meals, consider starting with one meal daily, where you commit fully to the practice. It could be breakfast, where you can start your day grounded and centered, or dinner, where it can serve as a peaceful transition from the busyness of your day. Use this meal as an opportunity to practice mindful eating techniques, turning them into habits that can eventually span across all your meals.

Additionally, involve your family or housemates in this practice. Share the principles of mindful eating and encourage everyone to participate. This makes the training more enjoyable and helps cultivate a supportive eating environment where everyone is engaged and present. It transforms mealtime from a routine to a shared ritual, enhancing the relational aspect of dining, which can be just as nourishing as the food on your plate.

Mindful eating is not a diet but a way to enhance your eating experiences and improve your digestion. It encourages a harmonious relationship with food and teaches you to value quality over quantity. By adopting mindful eating practices, you're not just feeding your body. You're nourishing your soul and fostering a calm, connected approach to eating that reverberates through your entire digestive system.

As we wrap up this exploration of how your lifestyle choices significantly impact your gut health, we see that it's not just about what you do occasionally but what you integrate consistently into your life. Each aspect supports your digestive health, from managing stress and ensuring adequate sleep to maintaining physical activity and proper hydration. Mindful eating is the cherry on top, turning every meal into an opportunity for enhancing digestive wellness and overall well-being.

In the next chapter, we'll explore how to manage specific challenges like dietary restrictions and food intolerances, ensuring your gut health journey is as smooth and enjoyable as possible. Let's continue to explore, learn, and grow in understanding this fascinating and essential aspect of our health.

UNLOCKING DIGESTIVE FREEDOM, WEIGHT WELLNESS, AND MENTAL CLARITY MADE EASY

Gut health is super important for your overall health. If you want better immunity, digestion, mental clarity, more energy, and balanced hormones, it's all about taking care of your gut. Your gut is like the command center for your health!

People who give without expecting anything back live longer, happier lives, and even make more money. So, during our time together, I'm going to try to give you the best information I can.

To make this happen, I have a question for you...

Would you help someone you've never met, even if you never got credit for it?

Who is this person, you ask? They are just like you. Or, at least, like you used to be. They are less experienced, wanting to make a difference, needing help, but not sure where to look.

Our mission is to make *The Beginner's Guide to Gut Health* accessible to everyone. Everything I do stems from that mission. And, the only way for me to accomplish that mission is by reaching...well...everyone.

This is where you come in. Most people do, in fact, judge a book by its cover (and its reviews). So here's my ask on behalf of anyone wanting to learn more about gut health and become healthier:

Please help that person by leaving this book a review.

Your gift costs no money and less than 60 seconds to make real, but it can change someone's life forever. Your review could help...

...one more small business provide for their community.
...one more entrepreneur support their family.
...one more employee get meaningful work.
...one more client transform their life.
...one more dream come true.

To get that 'feel good' feeling and help this person for real, all you have to do is...and it takes less than 60 seconds...

leave a review.

Simply scan the QR code below to leave your review:

If you feel good about helping someone learn about gut health, you are my kind of person. Welcome to the club. You're one of us.

I'm that much more excited to help you be more educated about the effects of our gut health and ways to improve it easier than you can possibly imagine. You'll love the lessons I'm about to share in the coming chapters.

Thank you from the bottom of my heart. Now, back to our regularly scheduled programming.

- Your biggest fan, Christina B. Kiser

P.S. - Fun fact: If you provide something of value to another person, it makes you more valuable to them. If you'd like to spread goodwill straight from another person who cares about gut health —and you believe this book will help them—send this book their way.

CHAPTER SIX

OVERCOMING COMMON GUT HEALTH CHALLENGES

I magine this: you're on a treasure hunt, but instead of searching for buried gold, you're on a quest for gut-nourishing foods that don't break the bank. You might think that eating for optimal gut health requires a wallet as robust as your digestive system ought to be, but let's bust that myth right now. Eating well for your gut doesn't have to mean splurging on exotic ingredients or shopping exclusively at high-end grocery stores. It's all about smart shopping, savvy planning, and knowing a trick or two to stretch those dollars.

6.1 AFFORDABLE, GUT-HEALTHY EATING

Budget-Friendly Foods: Your Gut's Best Friends

Let's kick things off with a list of wallet-friendly, gut-loving foods. Think of lentils, beans, oats, and bananas. These staples are inexpensive and packed with fiber, like a love letter to your microbiome. Then there's yogurt and kefir, which bring probiotics to the party without costing a fortune, especially if you opt for more extensive, generic brand containers. And let's remember frozen vegetables and fruits. They are often less expensive than their fresh counterparts and are picked at peak ripeness, locking in all the good nutrients.

Shopping for these items doesn't require a map. They can be found in any local supermarket. Incorporating them into your diet can be as simple as adding beans to a salad, swapping meat for lentils once a week, or starting your day with a bowl of oatmeal topped with frozen berries. Each meal becomes an opportunity to feed your gut the nutrients it needs without draining your wallet.

Shopping Strategies: Smart Tactics for the Budget-Conscious

Now, let's move on to the strategies that will turn you from a casual shopper into a savvy supermarket strategist. First, buying in bulk can significantly cut costs, especially for non-perishable items like rice, dried beans, and nuts. Think of it as stockpiling your gut health arsenal. Another strategy is to embrace seasonal produce. Vegetables and fruits are cheapest when they are in abundance, and they're also at their nutritional peak. You can visit local farmers' markets in the late hours for the best deals, as vendors are likely to discount produce rather than take it back home.

Another tip is to be flexible with your shopping list. If you go to the store with a meal plan but find that chicken is twice the price of turkey, be ready to pivot. This flexibility lets you take advantage of sales and discounts, keeping your gut and wallet full.

Cost-Effective Meal Planning: Maximize Your Meals without Minimizing Nutrients

Effective meal planning is like plotting your route before a road trip. It ensures you get to your destination efficiently without unnecessary stops or detours. Start by planning your meals around the budget-friendly foods listed earlier. Use sales flyers from local grocery stores to inspire your meal planning for the week—perhaps a discount on bell peppers could lead to a stuffed pepper dinner night.

Batch cooking is your friend here. Preparing large quantities of meals at once saves time and ingredients. Cook a big pot of chili or a hearty vegetable stew, then freeze into portions. You've got several meals ready and used up all your perishables before they could perish. It's a win-win.

Myths Around Cost: Debunking the Pricey Plate Perspective

Finally, let's tackle a pervasive myth: that healthy eating is prohibitively expensive. While it's true that some health-focused items can be pricey, essential nutrition, especially for gut health, doesn't have to be. It's more about how you shop and prepare food than where you shop. Beans, grains, seasonal produce, and bulk frozen goods offer the best nutritional bang for your buck.

Reflective Element: Budget Reflection Exercise

Take a moment to review your last grocery receipt. Which items were the most expensive? Could you swap any of these for a more budget-friendly, gut-healthy alternative? Next time you shop, challenge yourself to cut your grocery bill by 10% while filling your cart with nutritious foods that feed your microbiome. It's a practical exercise reinforcing the idea that economics can also mean nutrition.

By embracing these strategies and foods, you can nourish your gut without depleting your wallet. It's about making informed, mindful choices that benefit your digestive and financial health, proving that the two can go hand in hand.

6.2 QUICK AND SIMPLE GUT-HEALTHY RECIPES

Gut health is the unsung hero in our daily lives, influencing everything from our mood to our immune system. But let's be honest—between juggling work, family, and the occasional (or not-so-occasional) Netflix binge, who has the time to whip up complicated, gut-friendly meals? Fear not, because I've got your back with some quick and straightforward gut-healthy recipes that'll have you and your family's guts singing praises without chaining you to the kitchen.

Recipe Introduction: The Fast Lane to Flavorful Gut Health

Imagine this: recipes that are as easy to assemble as they benefit your gut. We're talking minimal ingredients and steps, but maximum flavor and gut benefits. These recipes use easily accessible ingredients that won't have you trekking across town to specialty stores. For instance, a smoothie that blends bananas, spinach, a scoop of Greek yogurt, and a dash of chia seeds can become a morning ritual that feels less like a chore and more like a treat. Or consider the magic of a one-tray bake—chop up some carrots, sweet potatoes, and chicken, toss them on a tray with olive oil and herbs, and let the oven do the work. It's about crafting meals that are so straightforward they practically make themselves.

Let's also chat about gut heroes like kimchi and sauerkraut. These fermented wonders can be intimidating if you're new to them but adding them to your meals can be as simple as topping your scrambled eggs with a spoonful of kimchi or throwing some sauerkraut into your salad for an extra crunch. These additions bring a zesty flavor to your meals and introduce beneficial probiotics to your diet, which are great for maintaining a healthy gut flora.

Meal Prep Tips: Your Strategy for Success

Efficient meal prep is your secret weapon for a healthier gut. It's all about making your kitchen work for you. Spend a couple of hours on a Sunday chopping veggies, cooking grains like quinoa or rice, and maybe roasting a chicken. Store these in the fridge, and you have a mix-and-match arsenal for quick meals throughout the week. Think bowls brimming with greens, grains, protein, and a dollop of fermented veggies—delicious, nutritious, and oh-so-easy to assemble.

Another tip is to embrace the power of the freezer. Soups and stews are perfect for making in large batches and then freezing in portions. Imagine coming home on a chilly evening to find a gut-friendly soup that needs a quick warm-up. It's like having a meal fairy godmother on standby. Cooking in batches means controlling what goes into your food and avoiding the excess sodium and preservatives often found in store-bought versions.

Diverse Meal Options: A World of Flavor at Your Fingertips

Diversity isn't just the spice of life. It's also a vital component of a gut-healthy diet. Different foods provide different nutrients and feed different beneficial bacteria in your gut. So, let's keep things interesting! How about starting with a Mediterranean Monday, where you serve a simple Greek salad with olives, cucumber, tomato, and feta, all tossed with olive oil and lemon? Then, take a trip to Mexico on Tuesday with a quick taco bowl featuring ground turkey, black beans, avocado, and a heap of leafy greens.

And for those who adore Asian flavors, a speedy stir-fry with plenty of ginger and garlic can do wonders for your gut health, thanks to these ingredients' anti-inflammatory properties. Use whatever veggies you have on hand, throw in some tofu or chicken, and you've got a gut-friendly meal that's also a feast for your taste buds. The key is to rotate your meals to include a variety of ingredients, ensuring that your gut gets a broad spectrum of nutrients.

Family-Friendly Meals: Everyone's Happy

Lastly, let's ensure the whole family can enjoy these meals. It's about finding that sweet spot where gut health meets palate pleasure. Take the humble spaghetti bolognese. Swap out regular pasta for a whole grain or legume-based alternative for an extra fiber boost, and add finely chopped mushrooms to the sauce for a dose of vitamin D. It's still the comforting classic everyone loves but tweaked for better gut health.

How about making pizza night more gut-friendly? A homemade pizza with a whole wheat base, topped with tomato sauce (rich in fiber and vitamin C), mozzarella, and a heap of vegetables like bell peppers and onions, can turn a guilty pleasure into a guilt- free delight. It's about making minor adjustments that won't cause a family uproar but will quietly improve everyone's gut health.

By incorporating these quick, simple, and delicious recipes and tips into your routine, you're feeding your family and fostering healthier, happier guts for everyone. And the best part? It doesn't require all your free time or a culinary degree—just the willingness to try some new tricks in the kitchen. Here's to gut health that fits seamlessly into your busy life, one tasty, nutritious meal at a time.

6.3 MANAGING GUT HEALTH ON THE GO

Ah, you are traveling! Maintaining gut health while hopping through time zones or exploring new cuisines can feel like trying to solve a Rubik's Cube blindfolded. Fear not! With a bit of foresight and a sprinkle of ingenuity, you can keep your gut happy, no matter how far your travels take you from home.

Travel Tips: Your Gut's Best Pal on the Road

Embarking on a journey doesn't mean your gut health has to take a back seat. Let's start with the basics: food packing. It's your first line of defense against the unpredictable culinary world that awaits you. Packing gut-friendly snacks like whole grain crackers, nuts, and high-fiber bars can be a lifesaver during long flights or road trips where healthy options are as rare as an empty middle seat on a budget airline. These snacks keep hunger at bay and ensure your gut microbes have the right fuel to thrive.

Choosing where and what to eat when dining out can often feel like navigating a minefield, especially when unfamiliar with the local cuisine. Opt for dishes that include components similar to those in your regular diet. For instance, if your gut is used to a fiber-rich diet, look for menu options rich in vegetables, whole grains, or legumes.

Don't shy away from asking the waiter about the ingredients—they're your allies in the quest to avoid unexpected digestive drama. It's about making informed choices that align with your gut health needs, even when miles away from your usual grocery store or kitchen.

Snack Ideas: Quick, Healthy, and Gut-Friendly

Snacking often gets a bad rap, but when you're on the go, it can be a gut-saver, especially with creativity and planning. Imagine transforming typical travel snacks into gut health powerhouses. For instance, mix your trail mix with nuts and seeds (like chia or flaxseed) and maybe some air-popped popcorn. This isn't just a snack; it's a fiber feast that keeps your gut microbes jubilant and your hunger at bay.

Another great option is to pack portable, non-perishable probiotic foods. Think probiotic yogurt drinks or even some types of cheese like Gouda, which are travel- friendly and offer the probiotic boost your gut craves. And let's remember fruits like apples, pears, or any other fiber-rich fruits that are easy to toss into your travel bag. These natural treats keep things sweet for your taste buds and gut bacteria.

Hydration While Traveling: Keeping the Flow

Staying hydrated is crucial, yet it's easy to neglect when caught up in travel. Your gut, much like your favorite houseplant, needs water to thrive. Dehydration can lead to digestive discomforts like constipation and bloating, turning your dream vacation into a not-so-pleasant memory. Always carry a reusable water bottle and fill it up at every opportunity. Many airports now have water refill stations, perfect for staying hydrated before a flight without buying overpriced bottled water.

Besides water, herbal teas are a fantastic hydration ally, with the added benefit of supporting digestion. Peppermint tea, for instance, can soothe your stomach and reduce bloating, making it a perfect travel companion. So, next time you pass by a coffee shop at the airport, consider opting for an herbal tea that hydrates and soothes your digestive system.

Navigating Restaurant Menus: A Gut-Friendly Guide

Eating out is integral to traveling, but it doesn't have to be a gut-wrenching experience. When scanning a menu, look for grilled, baked, or steamed dishes—cooking methods that typically use less oil and are gentler on your gut. Steer clear of overly creamy or fried dishes, which can be harder to digest, especially if your system isn't used to them.

Don't hesitate to ask for modifications. Most restaurants are more than willing to accommodate requests like dressing on the side or substituting a side of fries for a salad. It's about maintaining control over your eating, even in unfamiliar territory. And if you need clarification on a dish's ingredients or how it's prepared, a simple question can be the difference between a delightful meal and digestive distress.

Navigating your gut health while on the move isn't just about avoiding discomfort. It's about empowering yourself to enjoy your travels fully without the constant worry about your next meal. With these strategies, you're not just planning a trip - you're planning for your health, ensuring your vacation memories are full of adventure and free of avoidable digestive issues. So, pack your bags, grab your snacks, and set forth with the confidence that your gut health is cared for every step along the way.

6.4 NAVIGATING SOCIAL SITUATIONS WITH DIETARY RESTRICTIONS

When balancing dietary restrictions with a vibrant social life, every dinner invitation or office party can seem like a tightrope walk over a dietary dilemma. But fear not! With some finesse and planning, you can navigate these social waters without tipping the boat, keeping your gut health in check and your social life sparkling.

Effective Communication: Your Secret Weapon

Let's face it: explaining your dietary needs doesn't have to be as awkward as a blind date gone wrong. It's all about clear, confident communication. Calling ahead is okay when dining out or visiting a friend's place for dinner. A simple chat with your host or a quick word with the restaurant manager can make all the difference. Approach the conversation with positivity and gratitude: thank them for accommodating you and be concise about your dietary needs. It's not about listing your gut woes but providing a clear, practical rundown of what works for you. For instance, saying, "I find that gluten disrupts my digestion. Could we explore some gluten-free options?" is direct and helpful. This approach not only eases any potential stress on your part but also helps your hosts or servers be part of your solution, creating a more enjoyable experience for everyone involved.

Planning Ahead: A Smooth Strategy

Now, onto the art of planning. Your dietary wingman ensures you always have a game plan regardless of the social setting. Bring a dish that meets your nutritional criteria if you're headed to a potluck or a group event. This is your insurance policy—ensuring there's something on the table that you can enjoy without worry. Make something delicious and shareable, like a quinoa salad packed with veggies or a rich, gluten-free chocolate torte. Dishes like these won't just cater to your needs. They might steal the show, proving that dietary restrictions don't mean compromising on taste.

But what about impromptu gatherings or last-minute plans? Keeping a mental list of go-to restaurants that cater to your dietary requirements or packing a small snack can save the day. This proactive approach means you're never caught off guard and can still partake in spontaneous adventures without your gut paying the price.

Peer Support and Understanding: Building Your Team

While managing your diet on your terms is excellent, there's nothing quite like having a support squad. Whether it's family, friends, or coworkers, the people in your life can be a tremendous source of support. Don't shy away from sharing your experiences and what you've learned about managing your gut health. Often, people are curious and may only know how to help once you guide them.

Organize a cooking night where you and your friends make a gut-friendly meal together. It's fun to show them how delicious and satisfying such meals can be and give them a firsthand look at how you manage your dietary needs. Additionally, participating in or even starting a support group in person or online can connect you with others navigating similar challenges. These groups can be invaluable for sharing tips, recipes, and support. It's about creating a community that understands and uplifts each other, making managing dietary restrictions a shared, rather than solitary, journey.

Positive Focus: Emphasizing the Upsides

Lastly, focus on the positives when discussing your dietary restrictions with others. Getting caught up in the 'don't' and 'can't' is easy, but what about the benefits? Share how your diet has improved your health, energy levels, or mood. This shifts the conversation from one of restriction to one of enhancement. For instance, you might say, "Avoiding dairy has helped reduce my bloating and has surprisingly cleared up my skin!" This puts a positive spin on your dietary choices and helps others see your diet in a new light.

Navigating social situations with dietary restrictions doesn't have to be an arduous task. With clear communication, thoughtful planning, supportive relationships, and a focus on the positive aspects, you can maintain your social life and gut health, all while enjoying the rich tapestry of life's social offerings. Whether it's a wedding banquet, a work lunch, or a casual brunch, you're more than equipped to handle it with grace, confidence, and a bit of strategic planning. So go ahead, RSVP 'Yes' to that invite, and step out with the assurance that your gut health is as protected as your social calendar is packed.

6.5 WHEN TO CONSIDER SEEING A GUT HEALTH SPECIALIST

Sometimes, despite your best efforts with diet and lifestyle, your gut might still feel like it's throwing a perpetual tantrum. If you've been playing the role of both detective and doctor, but your digestive distress refuses to take a bow, it might be time to call in the professionals. Recognizing when to seek help can be the difference between enduring persistent discomfort and stepping onto the path of tailored, effective treatment.

So, what are the flashing neon signs that it's time to see a specialist? Persistent symptoms like chronic bloating, gas, diarrhea, constipation, or a combination can be your cue. If you find yourself popping antacids more often than popcorn for movie night, that's a signal. Given the gut-brain connection, unexplained weight changes, continuous fatigue, and even mood swings can also be rooted in gut issues. Your body sends you urgent emails: "Please pay attention to me - something is off!"

Regarding whom should be on your wellness team, gastroenterologists and nutritionists are the usual go-to professionals. Gastroenterologists specialize in the digestive system and its disorders. They're like gut whisperers, adept at diagnosing and treating conditions that affect your gastrointestinal (GI) tract. On the other hand, nutritionists can help you tweak your diet to alleviate symptoms and manage conditions through food, which is often a first-line therapy before escalating to more invasive treatments. Both professionals bring different skills and perspectives, making them invaluable in your quest for gut health.

Preparing for your visit is crucial. It's like prepping for a big exam —you'll perform better if you come equipped. Start a symptom diary now if you haven't already done so. Track what you eat, how it makes you feel, and any symptoms. Include any supplements or medications you use that can influence your gut health and treatment plan. Prepare questions in advance. Ask about diagnostic tests you might need, treatment options, and lifestyle changes you should consider. It's time to dig deep—don't leave wishing you had asked more questions.

Integrating professional advice with your ongoing personal health journey is like blending a new favorite smoothie recipe into your routine. It might shake things up, but it will enrich your wellness regimen. A healthcare professional can provide tailored advice based on your specific condition, which you can incorporate into your lifestyle with the adjustments you've already worked on. This holistic approach ensures you're not just putting a band-aid on the symptoms but are addressing underlying causes and contributing factors.

In this chapter, we've discussed the when, who, and how of turning to professionals for help with gut issues. Recognizing the signs, understanding the types of specialists available, preparing effectively for consultations, and integrating professional advice into your life all empower you to take control of your gut health confidently. Remember, seeking help is not a sign of defeat - it's an act of taking charge of your health and well-being.

As we close this chapter and look ahead, consider how the insights from professional consultations can be woven into the broader tapestry of your health practices. In the next chapter, we'll explore advanced topics in gut health, diving into emerging research and innovative treatments shaping the future of digestive wellness. Stay tuned because your gut health journey will get even more enjoyable.

CHAPTER SEVEN

THE GUT AND WOMEN'S HEALTH

P icture this: your gut and hormones are like an old married couple. They communicate constantly and influence each other's moods. Things can get complicated when they're not in sync. Understanding this relationship is crucial, especially for women, as it turns out that the ebb and flow of your hormones through different phases of your life—from menstrual cycles to menopause—can significantly impact your gut health and vice versa. It's a bi-directional relationship where each affects the state of the other—like a dance where sometimes the gut leads, and sometimes the hormones do.

7.1 HORMONES AND GUT HEALTH: UNDERSTANDING THE CONNECTION

Bi-Directional Relationship

Let's dive deeper into this dance between your hormones and gut health. It's essential to grasp that this isn't just about your gut causing mood swings or hormonal changes. It's also about how your hormonal balance can impact the well-being of your gut. For instance, many women experience changes in their digestive system at different stages of their menstrual cycle. Have you ever noticed that bloating feeling or your digestion seems slightly off during certain times of the month? That's your hormones playing a direct role in modulating your gut function. This modulation can lead to variations in how your body handles inflammation and even how it responds to the bacteria in your gut.

Estrogen and the Microbiome

Now, let's spotlight estrogen, an essential hormone that plays a starring role in this intricate dance. Estrogen has a profound impact on the makeup of your gut microbiome. Higher estrogen levels are generally associated with an increase in the microbiome's diversity, which is good because a diverse microbiome is resilient and better at withstanding and recovering from disruptions. This means when your estrogen levels are well-balanced, your gut is likely more varied and potentially healthier. However, during phases of life when estrogen levels fluctuate or drops, such as during the menstrual cycle or approaching menopause, there can be noticeable shifts in gut flora, which might explain some of the gastrointestinal discomforts experienced during these times.

Impact on Fertility and Menstrual Cycle

Speaking of menstrual cycles, did you know that your gut health can play a role in the regularity and health of your cycle? It's true. The gut influences levels of inflammation throughout your body, which can impact your hormones and thus your fertility and menstrual cycle regularity. A well-balanced gut can help manage inflammation, possibly leading to more regular cycles and positively impacting fertility. Attention to gut health might be as crucial as tracking ovulation for women trying to conceive.

Strategies for Hormonal Balance

So, how do you keep this complex system in balance? Let's talk strategy. Diet is monumental here. Foods rich in phytoestrogens, like flax, soy, and sesame seeds, can help modulate estrogen levels naturally. These foods mimic the effects of estrogen in your body, helping to balance levels. Fiber-rich foods also play a crucial role in eliminating excess hormones through the digestive process, thus preventing reabsorption.

Beyond diet, managing stress is another powerful tool. Stress can wreak havoc on your gut and hormonal balance, leading to a cascade of health issues. Regular stress- reduction techniques like yoga, meditation, or simple breathing exercises can help maintain hormonal balance and gut health.

Reflective Section: Hormonal Harmony Through Gut Health

Consider this your checkpoint. Reflect on your current diet and lifestyle: Are you feeding your gut the nutrients it needs to support a healthy hormone balance? How often do you engage in stress-reduction activities? This reflection isn't just about assessing and actively planning improvements. It could be tweaking your diet to include more phytoestrogen-rich foods, or it could be time for stress-reducing practices. Each small step is a step toward not just better gut health but better hormonal health, too.

Understanding and managing this relationship can improve health outcomes in the grand ballet of your body, where hormones and gut health are perennial dance partners. From easing menstrual irregularities to enhancing fertility and even smoothing the transition into menopause, the payoffs of nurturing this connection are profound and lasting. So, keep the dance going —nourish your gut, balance your hormones, and watch your health transform, one twirl and dip at a time.

7.2 GUT HEALTH DURING PREGNANCY AND POSTPARTUM

This period brings about significant shifts in your gut microbiome, which is as natural as the cravings for pickles dipped in peanut butter. But it's not just quirky food desires. These microbial changes play a critical role in your health and your baby's development. During pregnancy, your body becomes a finely tuned ecosystem, altering its microbial composition in ways that can influence everything from nutrient absorption to your immune system's functioning. These changes are believed to support the increased demands of pregnancy and prepare the body for delivery.

The role of gut health extends beyond just the mother. It's fascinating to consider that a mother's microbiome becomes the first encounter the newborn has with a world of bacteria, setting the stage for the infant's future gut health. This initial bacterial colonization is crucial, as it influences the baby's developing immune system and metabolism. Thus, maintaining a balanced and healthy gut during pregnancy isn't just about supporting your health - it's about giving your baby a head start in building a resilient microbiome. This is why consuming a diet rich in varied probiotics and prebiotics is akin to laying down a lush, green lawn where your baby's health can picnic for years.

Moving into the postpartum phase, the focus on gut health doesn't wane. Instead, it shifts into supporting recovery and adjusting to the new demands of motherhood. This period can be challenging, not just physically but emotionally, with the risk of postpartum depression looming as a serious concern for many new mothers. A well- balanced gut microbiome during this time can be a strong ally. Emerging research suggests that the gut-brain axis—yes, that intimate communication line between your digestive system and your mental state—plays a part in emotional well-being. A healthy gut can help mitigate the risk of postpartum depression, making foods rich in omega-3 fatty acids, fiber, and probiotics not just a dietary choice but a buffer against the emotional storms post-birth.

The nutritional needs during pregnancy and postpartum are like the fuel for this intricate operation. It's not just about eating more - it's about eating smart. Iron, for instance, is crucial due to increased blood volume and the needs of the growing fetus. Fiber is another non-negotiable, helping to keep the often-experienced constipation at bay. And let's not forget calcium and Vitamin D – essentials that support not just your bone health but that of your baby, too. Each meal is an opportunity to feed the gut bacteria that nourish and protect you and your child. It's about creating meals as rich in nutrients as they are in flavor, ensuring every bite contributes to a thriving microbial environment.

This focus on gut health throughout pregnancy and postpartum is less about following strict dietary protocols and more about listening to your body and responding with nourishment that supports you and your baby. It's a time of profound change and adaptation, and your gut is one of your most potent allies in navigating this beautiful, sometimes overwhelming, always life-changing landscape. So, as you prepare for and embrace motherhood, remember that taking care of your gut is a fundamental part of your overall health, helping ensure that you and your baby have the best start possible.

7.3 THE IMPACT OF MENOPAUSE ON GUT HEALTH

Ah, menopause is the time in a woman's life that's as unpredictable as a roulette wheel. Will it land on hot flashes, mood swings, or something unexpected today? But beyond these commonly talked-about symptoms, a less visible but equally significant change is happening: the shift in your gut microbiome during menopause. This change can play a sneaky role in some of the more frustrating aspects of menopause, like that mysterious weight gain that appears no matter how many kale smoothies you drink or miles you jog. As estrogen levels take a nosedive, the composition of your gut microbiota shifts, which can influence everything from your metabolism to your immune system. This shift can increase the body's fat storage and decrease metabolic rate, which might explain why maintaining your pre-menopause weight becomes a struggle.

But it's not just about weight. The changes in your microbiome also affect how your body handles inflammation, which can exacerbate other menopausal symptoms and contribute to health issues like cardiovascular disease and type 2 diabetes. It's like your body is suddenly playing by a new set of rules, and nobody gave you the manual. To combat this, focusing on a gut-friendly diet becomes even more crucial. This means feasting on fiber-rich foods, which can help manage weight by keeping you fuller for longer and promoting a healthy gut flora. Foods rich in phytoestrogens, such as soy products and flaxseeds, can also help mitigate hormonal fluctuations, as they provide a mild estrogenic effect in the body.

Transitioning smoothly from your gut's reaction to menopause, let's consider the critical connection between gut health and bone health during this phase of life. As estrogen levels drop, the risk of osteoporosis climbs—a worry for many women entering menopause. However, what's less commonly discussed is how gut health plays into this. A healthy gut aids calcium absorption, vital for maintaining strong bones. However, this absorption can be compromised when the microbiome is out of balance. Incorporating foods high in calcium and vitamin D strengthens this link. Think beyond dairy: leafy greens, almonds, and fortified plant milks are excellent allies.

Pairing these with probiotic-rich foods like yogurt and kefir can help enhance calcium absorption, making it a dynamic duo for keeping your bones as sturdy as your resolve.

Now, while adjusting your diet is a powerful tool, it's not the only lever you should pull. Lifestyle interventions play a massive role in managing the impact of menopause on both your gut health and overall well-being. Regular physical activity, for instance, can help offset weight gain, reduce stress, and improve sleep—all of which can help maintain a healthier gut. Activities like yoga and Pilates keep you fit and focus on core strength, which is beneficial for supporting back health and overall posture, reducing the risk of fractures as bone density decreases. Moreover, regular physical activity can enhance the diversity of your gut microbiome, which is linked to better health outcomes overall.

Creating a routine with mindfulness or relaxation practices can also significantly impact your menopausal experience. Stress is a notorious aggravator of menopausal symptoms and can negatively affect gut health, leading to a vicious cycle of discomfort and anxiety. Stress-reduction techniques such as meditation, deep-breathing exercises, or even time in nature can help soothe your mind and gut. It's about creating a holistic approach to this new stage in life. Embracing changes with strategies that support your body's new needs.

Navigating menopause with an eye on gut health offers a pathway to mitigating some of the less pleasant aspects of this transition. By understanding the interplay between your microbiome, dietary needs, and lifestyle choices, you can step into this phase with resilience and a plan that supports vitality, health, and continued joy in your body's journey. So, as you adjust to the new rhythms of your life, remember that your gut is critical to finding balance and well-being on this ride.

7.4 MANAGING PMS AND CRAMPS THROUGH GUT HEALTH

When it feels like your body's monthly memo is to turn your life upside-down with PMS and cramps, consider tuning into the gut-brain-hormone axis, a fascinating network that could be the key to easing those tumultuous times. This complex communication system between your gut, brain, and hormonal fluctuations doesn't just exist to complicate things - it offers a pathway to potential relief. Understanding this connection can be a game-changer in managing PMS symptoms. It's like finding out there's a shortcut in your daily commute that avoids all the traffic jams—it's empowering and can make the journey a lot more pleasant.

Each month, as your body prepares for the potential of pregnancy, hormones ebb and flow, creating the physical and emotional symptoms of PMS. But here's where it gets interesting: your gut influences these hormonal tides through interactions with your brain and your body's endocrine system. For example, serotonin, a key mood regulator produced primarily in your gut, can fluctuate during your menstrual cycle, impacting your mood and gut function. This can lead to those all-too-familiar cravings and mood swings, as well as bloating and digestive discomfort. By supporting gut health, you're essentially helping to stabilize the production and function of serotonin and other hormones involved in PMS, which can help smooth out some of the monthly turbulence.

Now, let's talk about the role of diet, particularly anti-inflammatory foods, in managing PMS and cramps. Foods rich in omega-3 fatty acids, like salmon, flaxseeds, and walnuts, are excellent for this. They help reduce the production of prostaglandins, chemicals that can cause heavy cramping and inflammation. It's similar to turning down the volume on a loudspeaker, blaring out discomfort signals. Incorporating more magnesium-rich foods such as spinach, pumpkin seeds, and dark chocolate (yes, your chocolate cravings are justified!) can also help relax your muscles, reducing cramp severity. Then there are the fiber-rich foods like fruits, vegetables, and whole grains that keep your digestion smooth and help regulate blood sugar levels, curbing those mood swings and irritability that can come with PMS.

Probiotics, too, deserve a spotlight for their role in this monthly drama. Specific strains like Lactobacillus acidophilus and Bifidobacterium bifidum can be beneficial. These probiotics help maintain a balanced gut microbiome, which is crucial because a disrupted gut can send signals that exacerbate hormonal imbalances and PMS symptoms. Regularly including probiotic-rich foods like yogurt, kefir, and sauerkraut in your diet or taking a high-quality probiotic supplement can help manage the microbial community in your gut, promoting overall hormonal balance and potentially easing those PMS blues.

Stress management is another critical piece of the puzzle. High stress can aggravate PMS symptoms, turning what might be a manageable tide of discomfort into a tsunami of emotional and physical pain. Techniques like mindfulness meditation, guided imagery, and progressive muscle relaxation can be powerful tools. These practices not only reduce stress but can also decrease the perception of pain, making them a double-edged sword against PMS. Regularly engaging in these activities can help recalibrate your body's stress response, potentially reducing the severity of PMS symptoms. It's like installing a sophisticated security system in your home - it doesn't stop the outside world from being chaotic, but it does help keep the chaos from overwhelming your personal space.

In this dance of hormones, gut health, and brain function, every step you take towards understanding and supporting your body's interconnected systems brings you closer to reclaiming your well-being during PMS. By embracing a diet rich in anti- inflammatory foods, nurturing your gut with probiotics, and managing stress, you create a stronger foundation to endure your menstrual cycle and thrive.

As we wrap up this exploration into the gut's influence on PMS and cramps, remember that your body is an intricate and dynamic system. The strategies discussed here are not just about alleviating symptoms but are part of a holistic approach to your health.

They offer a way to harmonize your body's natural rhythms with your lifestyle, transforming what can be a monthly ordeal into a more balanced, manageable experience. In the next chapter, we'll delve deeper into the fascinating world of the microbiome, uncovering more about its profound impacts on women's health and overall human health and disease.

CHAPTER EIGHT

MENTAL HEALTH AND THE MICROBIOME

Have you ever wondered if your gut might be the wizard behind the curtain of your mood swings or why, on some days, you feel like you're on a rollercoaster ride of emotions without even stepping into an amusement park? Well, strap in and let me unravel a tale as intriguing as any mystery novel: the complex relationship between your gut health and mental well-being.

8.1 ANXIETY, DEPRESSION, AND THE GUT: WHAT'S THE LINK?

Gut-Brain Axis Overview

Picture this: your gut and brain are like old college roommates who've kept in touch over the years through a direct hotline. This hotline is known as the gut-brain axis, an intricate communication network involving nerves, hormones, and immune system messengers that send updates back and forth. If your gut is feeling under the weather or flourishing, you can bet your brain will hear about it. This channel is why when your gut microbiome—the diverse community of microorganisms residing in your digestive tract—is out of balance, it might just manifest as mood swings, anxiety, or even symptoms of depression. It's less about the mystical "gut feelings" and more about biological signals directly impacting your brain's chemistry and function.

Neurotransmitter Production

Now, let's talk about when you feel a sudden surge of happiness after a good meal or a wave of calmness with comfort food. There's science behind that! Your gut microbes are like tiny chemists, concocting a variety of neurotransmitters—the body's natural chemical messengers. Serotonin, famously known as the 'feel-good' hormone, is predominantly produced in the gut. Yes, that's right, not just in the brain! This neurotransmitter plays a pivotal role in regulating mood, anxiety, and happiness. Similarly, the gut produces dopamine, another mood regulator controlling the brain's reward and pleasure centers. So, essentially, a well-balanced gut microbiome can mean better production and regulation of these crucial mood influencers, leading to a more stable emotional state.

Inflammation and Mental Health

But there's a plot twist: inflammation, the body's response to injury or attack, can turn this story sour. When the gut is inflamed —often due to poor diet, stress, or pathogens—it can increase systemic inflammation. This is not just about a stomachache or indigestion. This inflammation can also be a party crasher for your brain. It has been linked to an increased risk of mood disorders, including depression and anxiety. Essentially, if your gut is on fire, it might be fanning the flames of mood swings and other mental health issues.

Evidence-Based Research

The plot thickens with a growing body of research supporting these connections. Recent studies have illuminated the gut microbiome's profound impact on mental health. For instance, certain probiotics known as 'psychobiotics' have shown potential in alleviating symptoms of anxiety and depression by influencing the gut-brain axis.

These findings open up exciting avenues for therapeutic approaches targeting the gut microbiome to treat or manage mental health disorders. It's like discovering a new, less invasive way to calm the stormy seas of the mind through the gentle manipulation of the gut.

Reflective Section: Mind Your Gut

So, as you digest this information (pun intended!), consider your gut health. Could there be a link between those days you feel down and your gut's well-being?

Reflecting on your diet, stress levels, and overall lifestyle could provide insights into how your gut might influence your mental health. And remember, while it's not a magic bullet, maintaining a healthy and balanced gut microbiome could be a key player in your journey toward optimal mental wellness. It's about making choices that nourish not just your body but also your mind.

In this intricate dance between your gut and your brain, every meal, every stressor, and every lifestyle choice plays a part. By understanding and nurturing this connection, you empower yourself with one more strategy to enhance your mental health and quality of life. So next time you're about to indulge in that fiber-rich salad or consider skipping that meditation session, remember the profound impact such actions might have on your mental canvas. Your gut, your brain, and indeed, your entire being might thank you for it.

8.2 PROBIOTICS AS A PATHWAY TO MENTAL CLARITY

Have you ever considered that those tiny, bustling communities of bacteria thriving in your gut could be your allies in clearing the mental fog? Welcome to the fascinating world of psychobiotics, a charming term that might sound like something out of a sci-fi novel but is very much a part of cutting-edge mental health research. Psychobiotics are specific types of probiotics, those friendly bacteria you often hear touted for their digestive benefits, which have shown promise in boosting mental health. These microscopic marvels do more than aid digestion - they could be critical players in sharpening your mind and elevating your mood.

The intrigue around psychobiotics stems from their potential to alter brain function through the gut-brain axis—the communication highway between your gut and brain. It's like having a direct line from your gut to your mental well-being, where these tiny organisms send chemical messages that can positively affect your mood and cognitive functions. For example, certain strains of probiotics are known to produce neurotransmitters, like GABA and serotonin, which are directly involved in regulating anxiety and depression. This means that the right balance of gut bacteria could help increase the levels of these feel-good chemicals in your brain, giving you a natural boost in combating mood disorders.

Recent clinical studies have provided a peek into this potential, showing promising results in the use of specific probiotic strains to treat symptoms of depression and anxiety. In one study, participants taking a probiotic supplement containing Lactobacillus (L.) helveticus and Bifidobacterium (B.) long reported significant reductions in stress and anxiety compared to those taking a placebo. Another research experiment focused on Lactobacillus plantarum strain PS128, showing it altered brain activity associated with emotional responses and reduced anxiety-like behaviors in individuals without mood disorders. These studies suggest that psychobiotics could one day be part of routine treatment plans for mental health issues, offering a low-side-effect alternative to traditional pharmaceuticals.

Now, before you rush off to stock your fridge with all the yogurt and sauerkraut you can find, let's talk about how to choose wisely and use these probiotics for mental health.

Not all probiotics are created equal, especially regarding their effects on mental health. The strain and the dosage matter immensely. For instance, the strains mentioned earlier, L. helveticus and B. longum, have explicitly been studied for their effects on reducing stress and anxiety. When selecting a probiotic supplement, look for products that specify the strains used and provide information on the number of living organisms per dose, usually listed as colony-forming units (CFUs). A daily dose of around 10 billion CFUs is generally recommended, but this can vary based on the specific strains and the product.

Incorporating psychobiotics into your routine doesn't have to be a chore. Many probiotic-rich foods, such as kefir, kombucha, and certain cheeses, are delicious and a great way to support your mental health. If you opt for a supplement, consider it part of your morning routine to help establish a consistent habit. Remember, while psychobiotics are a thrilling area of development in mental health and wellness, they're most effective when used as part of a broader approach to health that includes a balanced diet, regular exercise, and proper sleep—all crucial for optimal mental well-being.

So, as you continue to navigate the complex world of mental health, keep in mind the potential of psychobiotics as a tool in your arsenal for clarity and wellness. With ongoing research and a thoughtful approach to incorporating these beneficial bacteria into your life, you're on your way to a healthier gut and a more transparent, vibrant mind.

8.3 GUT HEALTH STRATEGIES FOR STRESS REDUCTION

Stress—it's like that uninvited guest who not only crashes your party but also makes a mess in your kitchen, and oh, your gut is the kitchen in this metaphor. Chronic stress doesn't just frazzle your brain, it throws a wrench in the delicate ecosystem of your gut microbiome. Under stress, your body ramps up the production of stress hormones like cortisol, which can throw your gut bacteria out of whack, reducing the diversity and number of those friendly microbes that keep your digestive system running smoothly. This disruption can lead to all sorts of fun (read: not fun at all) issues like inflammation, increased susceptibility to infections, and even changes in gut motility—

yes, that means both constipation and the dreaded diarrhea. But fear not, because just as your lifestyle can feed into this cycle of stress and gut chaos, it can also be your most potent weapon in breaking it.

Your diet is one of your most delicious tools in this battle against stress. What you put on your plate can profoundly influence your stress levels and gut health. Let's start with a fan favorite—fiber. Found in fruits, vegetables, whole grains, and legumes, fiber isn't just good for keeping things moving in your digestive tract, it also feeds those beneficial gut bacteria. These microbes, in turn, produce short-chain fatty acids that have a calming effect on your gut lining and may help reduce the inflammation that stress can cause. And let's not forget about fermented foods like yogurt, kefir, and sauerkraut. These probiotic-rich foods help bolster your gut's army of good bacteria, which can be depleted by constant stress.

But it's not just about adding things to your diet - it's also about what to limit. High- sugar and high-fat foods might be your go-to when stressed (hello, ice cream), but they can be like throwing gasoline on a fire regarding your gut health. These foods can promote the growth of less-friendly bacteria and yeasts, exacerbating gut dysbiosis and inflammation, so while that pint of double fudge ripple might seem like a good idea at the moment, your gut (and your stress levels) will thank you if you reach for a bowl of mixed berries or a dark chocolate square instead.

Shifting gears from what you eat to how you live, regular exercise is another effective strategy for both managing stress and supporting your gut health. Physical activity helps reduce levels of the body's stress hormones, such as adrenaline and cortisol and stimulates the production of endorphins, your brain's feel-good neurotransmitters. And here's a fun fact: regular exercise can also increase the diversity of your gut microbiome, which is linked to better overall health and improved mood regulation.

Whether it's a brisk walk, a yoga session, or a dance party in your living room, moving your body can be a powerful way to de-stress and support your gut.

Lastly, let's talk about the superhero duo of stress reduction: mindfulness and meditation. These practices are like a spa day for your brain and gut. Mindfulness or meditation can help decrease the body's stress response and bring about a sense of calm and focus, often lost when stress runs rampant. These practices have been shown to reduce symptoms of anxiety and depression, improve focus, and decrease cortisol levels, which can help rebalance your gut microbiome. Whether through guided meditation sessions, mindful breathing exercises, or simply taking a few moments each day to be present with your thoughts, incorporating mindfulness into your routine can help fortify your mental and gut health against the impacts of stress.

So, there you have it—a toolkit for tackling stress that helps calm your mind and soothes your gut. By embracing a diet rich in fiber and probiotics, engaging in regular physical activity, and incorporating mindfulness and meditation into your routine, you're managing stress and cultivating a gut environment that can stand firm against the chaos of daily life. Think of these strategies as your wellness regimen, designed to keep your mental and gut health in check, allowing you to navigate life's stresses with a bit more ease and much more health.

8.4 THE ROLE OF DIET IN MANAGING MOOD DISORDERS

Welcome to the intriguing world of nutritional psychiatry, where your dinner plate might hold the key to your mood. This relatively new field explores how what you eat directly affects your brain's structure, chemistry, physiology, mood, and mental health. Think of it as the culinary science of the mind. It's a fascinating exploration that has begun to unravel how specific diets can act like slow-release medication for your mood without the side effects often associated with traditional drugs.

One of the superheroes of this dietary approach is the anti-inflammatory diet. This isn't just about soothing sore muscles or calming chronic skin conditions- it's also about cooling down inflammation in your brain. Chronic inflammation is increasingly linked to mood disorders such as depression and anxiety. By adopting an anti-inflammatory diet, you're essentially putting out fires in your brain that can lead to or exacerbate these conditions. This diet emphasizes foods rich in antioxidants, like berries and leafy greens, which combat free radicals and reduce oxidative stress, a key promoter of inflammation. It also includes hearty helpings of whole grains and fatty fish, nuts, and seeds, all of which fight inflammation. The idea is to create a meal plan that not only delights your taste buds but also keeps inflammation— and thus mood disorders—at bay.

Now, let's dive deeper into the waters of omega-3 fatty acids, known for their role in brain health and mood regulation. These fats are the brain's best friends. They help build and repair brain cells and are potent anti-inflammatory agents. Omega-3s are abundant in fatty fish like salmon, mackerel, and sardines, which should be on your menu at least a couple of times a week. If you're not a fan of fish, consider flaxseeds, chia seeds, or walnuts, which are also excellent sources. Regular intake of these omega-3 powerhouses can help enhance the fluidity of your brain's cell membranes, making it easier for mood-related neurotransmitters like serotonin and dopamine to dance across neural synapses. The result? A smoother mood landscape without the peaks and troughs.

However, while adding certain foods can support mental health, removing others can be equally beneficial. Processed foods, high in sugar and unhealthy fats, are like the villains of this story. They often cause a rapid spike and subsequent crash in blood sugar levels, which can lead to mood swings and irritability. Moreover, these foods can aggravate inflammation and disrupt the delicate balance of your gut microbiome, further impacting your mental health. Artificial additives, often abundant in processed foods, can also interfere with brain function and mood regulation. The strategy here is simple: steer clear of foods that act as kindling for mood disorders. Instead, focus on fresh, whole foods that nourish your body and brain.

Navigating the complex interplay of diet and mood means not just feeding your stomach. You're nourishing your brain and nurturing your mental health. You're taking proactive steps toward a happier, healthier mind by choosing anti-inflammatory foods rich in omega-3s and avoiding processed sugar-laden products. It's a form of self-care that's as delicious as beneficial. So next time you plan your meals, think of your kitchen as your pharmacy, where every dish is a dose of mood medicine.

As we wrap up this chapter, remember that your fork is a powerful tool—not just for feeding your body but for stabilizing and uplifting your mood. The principles of nutritional psychiatry can guide you in choosing foods that support mental wellness and creating a diet that's as good for your brain as it is for your taste buds. In the next chapter, we'll explore advanced gut health topics, digging deeper into emerging research and innovative treatments highlighting the gut's critical role in overall health and disease. Stay tuned because the journey through your body's inner ecosystem will get even more profound.

CHAPTER NINE

CREATING YOUR GUT HEALTH SUPPORT SYSTEM

This chapter is about building your support system, an essential lifeline that can make all the difference in navigating the sometimes-turbulent waters of gut health. Whether finding allies online, communicating effectively with loved ones, or connecting with knowledgeable healthcare providers, think of this as assembling your dream team. Each player brings something unique, from emotional support to expert advice, creating a holistic network that empowers you to take control of your gut health with confidence and camaraderie.

9.1 LEVERAGING ONLINE COMMUNITIES FOR SUPPORT

Virtual Support Networks

In the digital age, the world is literally at our fingertips, and this includes a vast array of online communities where you can find camaraderie and support for your gut health issues. These virtual platforms range from specialized forums and Facebook groups to subreddits on topics like probiotics, IBS, or the low-FODMAP diet. Here, you can connect with people who are in the same boat, sharing not just woes but also wins.

Think of these platforms as your 24/7 support group, where you can ask questions at midnight or share a breakthrough at dawn without waiting for the doctor's office to open.

Benefits of Online Communities

The charm of these online communities lies in their diversity and accessibility. Here, you can interact anonymously, which can be a massive relief if you're starting to navigate sensitive health issues and aren't quite ready to share your story with the world. This anonymity also encourages a more open exchange of information and experiences, allowing you to gather genuine insights and varied perspectives.

Moreover, these communities are buzzing hubs of activity at all hours, providing support and answers when needed, breaking the limitations of time zones and geography.

Finding the Right Fit

However, not all communities are created equal, and finding the right fit is critical to making your online experience positive and productive. Start by identifying forums that align with your specific gut health concerns. Look for communities that foster a supportive and respectful environment—places where misinformation is corrected, questions are welcomed, and victories are celebrated. It's also wise to observe the community's interactions before diving in. A promising sign is active moderation and a clear set of rules that promote constructive communication.

Safe Engagement Practices

While these communities offer numerous benefits, navigating them wisely is crucial. Always protect your privacy by not sharing personal information like your address or phone number. Be cautious about taking medical advice from non-professionals. While the support is invaluable, treatment and diagnosis should still be left to healthcare professionals. Additionally, I learned to distinguish between anecdotal experiences and evidence-based information. A helpful strategy is to look for repeated patterns or advice corroborated by reputable sources. This discernment makes you a savvy consumer of information, ensuring you benefit from the community without falling prey to the common pitfalls of online interactions.

Interactive Element: Reflection Section

Take a moment to reflect on your current support systems for your gut health. How diverse is your support network? Are you leveraging online communities to their full potential? Consider jotting down what you currently appreciate in these interactions and what you feel is lacking. This reflection can guide you in seeking out new groups or engaging differently in existing ones to enhance your support system effectively.

In this interconnected world, remember that you are not alone in your quest for better gut health. Online communities offer a unique and powerful resource for connection, information, and support, helping you navigate your health journey with an army of allies. Choosing the right communities and engaging with them wisely enriches your support system with collective knowledge and empathy, making the path to wellness a shared and more enjoyable adventure.

9.2 COMMUNICATING YOUR NEEDS TO FRIENDS AND FAMILY

When discussing gut health with your friends and family, it might feel like you're trying to explain why you're bringing a salad to a pizza party. But here's the scoop: opening up about your gut health isn't just about food choices - it's about inviting those closest to you into a critical aspect of your well-being. Initiating these conversations can sometimes feel as delicate as navigating a minefield, mainly when dietary changes affect social traditions and shared meals. However, articulating your needs clearly and sincerely can transform these interactions from potential conflicts into opportunities for deeper understanding and support.

Starting these discussions requires a blend of honesty and sensitivity. Begin by choosing a comfortable setting free of distractions and stress, where you can speak openly. It's helpful to communicate the 'what' of your gut health needs and the 'why.' Explain how certain foods impact your well-being, perhaps causing discomfort or flare- ups, and clarify why this matters. It's not just about the physical symptoms but how they affect your energy levels, mood, and enjoyment. When others understand gut health's profound impact on your overall quality of life, they're more likely to offer support instead of resistance.

Setting boundaries is also crucial, especially in social eating situations - often minefields of temptation and misunderstanding. It's okay to say no to grandma's famous lasagna if it wreaks havoc on your gut. Setting these boundaries kindly but firmly helps prevent discomfort and awkwardness at the dining table. It also teaches others to respect your health decisions, essential in maintaining your well-being and harmonious relationships. Try framing your dietary needs positively, focusing on what you can eat and enjoy rather than listing forbidden foods. This approach eases the conversation and invites others to explore and enjoy your dietary world without feeling it's about restrictions.

Sharing educational resources can also enrich these conversations. Sometimes, a well- chosen article, book, or even a documentary can explain aspects of gut health more eloquently or comprehensively than you might in casual chatter. These resources can provide a scientific or holistic view of why specific dietary changes are crucial, which might be more convincing for the skeptically minded family member. They also offer a broader context that your explanation might lack, showing that your dietary choices are not just personal whims but part of more comprehensive, well-researched strategies for better health.

Lastly, consider the power of seeking and accepting emotional support from your loved ones. Managing your diet and health routines solo is one thing, but having a support system can significantly lighten the emotional load. Whether it's having someone to talk to after a tough day of managing symptoms or celebrating a small victory in your health journey, these moments of sharing can strengthen your relationships and provide immense comfort and motivation. Encourage your loved ones to ask questions and share their feelings about your health journey. This two-way communication can foster empathy and understanding, making your support system robust and responsive.

Navigating gut health is not just a personal affair - it involves your community. Especially those closest to you. By communicating openly, setting clear boundaries, sharing informative resources, and fostering emotional connections, you can create a supportive environment that bolsters your efforts to manage your gut health. This approach doesn't just benefit you. It enriches your relationships, turning what might be a source of tension into a testament to mutual care and respect.

9.3 FINDING THE RIGHT HEALTHCARE PROVIDERS FOR GUT HEALTH

Selecting the right healthcare provider for gut health is akin to choosing the right chef for a five-star dining experience—finding someone who can blend the right ingredients (knowledge, experience, and care approach) to create the perfect recipe for your well- being. When embarking on this selection, it's essential to consider a blend of qualifications, treatment approaches, and patient feedback. A provider's credentials should include medical degrees and specialized training in gastroenterology or a related field.

However, degrees are just the starter dish. Dive deeper by exploring their treatment philosophies. Are they advocates of a purely conventional approach, or do they value integrative practices that include nutritional therapy and lifestyle changes?

Patient reviews can show how effectively a provider implements their approach. These reviews often highlight the provider's ability to listen and respond to patient concerns, a crucial ingredient in the care process that can significantly affect outcomes.

Embracing an integrative health approach can dramatically enhance the management of your gut health. This holistic strategy goes beyond merely prescribing medication to alleviate symptoms, focusing instead on identifying and treating the root causes of gut disorders, which often involve a combination of factors including diet, psychological stress, and physical health. Integrative medicine may include conventional pharmaceuticals as needed, but it also incorporates nutritional counseling, stress reduction techniques, physical therapy, and even alternative practices like acupuncture or herbal medicine. This blend ensures that all bases are covered, providing a more comprehensive treatment plan tailored to your unique needs and lifestyle.

Building a multidisciplinary healthcare team is another vital step in optimizing gut health management. Consider this team your health boardroom, with specialists from diverse fields crafting a holistic strategy to tackle your gut health issues. A gastroenterologist can diagnose and treat conditions directly related to gut health, while a nutritionist can provide invaluable insights into how your diet influences your symptoms and overall health. Including a mental health professional can also be beneficial, especially since the gut-brain connection plays a significant role in digestive health. Each professional brings a unique perspective, ensuring that all aspects of your health are considered and addressed. This collaborative approach increases the likelihood of successful treatment and provides a support system that empowers you to control your health journey actively.

Effective communication with your healthcare providers is the cornerstone of receiving optimal care. Discussing your symptoms and concerns as openly and in detail as possible is essential. Prepare for appointments by jotting down any symptoms, dietary habits, stress levels, and even your emotional state, as all these can influence gut health. During consultations, ask questions to clarify doubts and discuss potential treatment options and their side effects or benefits. It's also wise to discuss any research or alternative treatments you're considering. Remember, a good healthcare provider should listen and engage with you to develop a treatment plan that respects your views and comfort levels. This open dialogue ensures that you are fully informed and comfortable with your healthcare decisions, ultimately leading to better treatment outcomes and a more satisfying healthcare experience.

By taking the time to carefully select your healthcare providers, advocate for an integrative approach, build a comprehensive team, and communicate effectively, you equip yourself with a robust support system tailored to manage and improve your gut health. This proactive approach enhances your ability to cope with gut health issues. It is crucial to your overall health and well-being, ensuring you receive the most effective and personalized care possible.

9.4 THE POWER OF SHARING YOUR GUT HEALTH STORY

When you first start navigating the choppy waters of gut health issues, it can feel like you're adrift alone in a vast ocean. But here's a beacon of hope: sharing your personal experiences can light your way and illuminate the paths for others sailing similar seas.

Telling your story isn't just about unburdening yourself or broadcasting your life. It's a powerful act of community building and self-discovery that can profoundly impact both the teller and the listener.

Imagine the ripple effect of dropping your story like a pebble into the vast internet lake or through conversations. Each ripple reaches out, touches others, and provides something to relate to, learn from, or be inspired by. Whether through a blog post detailing your trial-and-error experiences with different diets, a heartfelt Instagram caption about a particularly challenging day, or an engaging talk at a local community center, these shared narratives foster a sense of connection and understanding. They transform personal struggles into communal waypoints - markers that guide and encourage others in their health quests.

Platforms like personal blogs, social media pages, and even YouTube channels have become modern-day campfires where we gather to share our tales of woes and wins in managing gut health. These platforms offer space to vocalize your journey and invite feedback, discussion, and support from a global audience. This interaction often creates a dynamic space where people feel less isolated in their struggles and more empowered to take action. Moreover, speaking at health seminars or workshops can be incredibly fulfilling for those who prefer live interaction. It raises awareness and positions you as a beacon of hope and practical advice for others.

The impact of sharing your gut health saga extends beyond just offering hope and information. It profoundly affects those in the early, often confusing stages of their gut health management. Your story could be the lifeline they need for someone discovering that they are not alone in experiencing bizarre symptoms or feeling overwhelmed by dietary changes. It reassures them that others have navigated these tricky waters and found ways to manage or thrive despite the challenges. This sense of community and belonging can be tremendously comforting and transform the journey from a solitary trek to a shared expedition.

Reflecting on and articulating your gut health experiences can also significantly enhance your understanding of your health. This reflective process often brings clarity, helping you see patterns or insights not apparent in discomfort or stress. It encourages mindfulness and proactive management, where you are more attuned to your body's needs and responses. Moreover, it can spur you to continue researching, experimenting, and learning about gut health, driving an ongoing cycle of self-improvement and advocacy.

In essence, sharing your story is about knitting a tapestry of experiences that enriches your understanding and contributes to a larger narrative of health and wellness. It's about creating a dialogue that informs and transforms, fostering a community where support and information flow freely. As you move forward, remember that each chapter of your health story you share does more than chronicle your journey. It paves the way for conversations, connections, and changes that can resonate far beyond your immediate circle.

As this chapter closes, think of it not as an ending but as an invitation to continue exploring, sharing, and growing in the vast, interconnected world of gut health. Your story is a powerful tool in this adventure that can inspire, guide, and connect, making the journey less daunting and more doable for everyone involved. So, as we turn the page to the next chapter, carry forward the spirit of sharing and community, for in the stories we tell, we find healing and hope for ourselves and others.

CHAPTER TEN

ADVANCED GUT HEALTH
TOPICS

I magine standing on the edge of a new frontier, not of uncharted territories on a map, but of the vast and mysterious landscape within you—your gut. In this chapter, we're donning our explorer's hats (metaphorically speaking) and diving into the thrilling future of gut health. With technologies that sound like they belong in a science fiction novel and therapies that could revolutionize how we treat many conditions, the horizon is buzzing with potential. So, let's embark on this adventure together, discovering how the latest breakthroughs and cutting-edge research are setting the stage for a gut health revolution.

10.1 THE FUTURE OF GUT HEALTH: EMERGING RESEARCH

Cutting-Edge Studies

The realm of gut health is experiencing a renaissance fueled by groundbreaking research reshaping our understanding of this complex system. One of the most dazzling stars in this galaxy of new knowledge is the study of microbiome mapping. Think of it as creating a detailed Google map of the bacterial universe inside your gut. This research reveals not just who's there in terms of bacteria but also what they're doing, how they interact, and their impact on everything from your metabolism to your mood. Fascinating is the gut-brain axis research, which uncovers how these microscopic inhabitants can communicate with your brain.

Technological Advances

As we venture further into the future, technology is setting a breathtaking pace. Innovations in gut health diagnostics and treatments are emerging faster than pop-up ads in a browser. For instance, imagine swallowing a tiny, pill-sized camera that can take thousands of pictures of your gut's interior as it travels through your digestive system. This capsule endoscopy is not just futuristic fun - it's a powerful tool that makes finding and treating gut issues easier and less invasive. Then there's the development of intelligent toilets—yes, you heard that right—that could analyze your waste in your bathroom, providing real-time data on your gut health. These technologies are turning the stuff of sci-fi into everyday tools that could vastly improve how we monitor and manage our gut health.

Potential Therapies

Hold onto your hats because the therapy advancements are where things get wild. Fecal microbiota transplants (FMT) might sound a bit... well, icky. Still, they're proving to be a game-changer in treating conditions like Clostridioides difficile infection, which can cause severe diarrhea and more serious intestinal conditions. This procedure involves transferring stool from a healthy donor into a patient's intestinal tract to restore a healthy microbial balance. Then there's the burgeoning field of personalized probiotics, which could one day allow us to customize bacterial supplements precisely to our unique gut flora needs, like mixing a personal smoothie that caters to your nutritional cravings.

The Role of Genetics

Our exploration is the genetic frontier—how our DNA influences gut health. With advances in genetic testing, we're beginning to understand that the interplay between our genes and gut bacteria is critical in everything from our susceptibility to infections to our response to specific diets. This knowledge heralds a move towards more personalized health strategies, where treatments and dietary recommendations can be tailored to your genetic makeup, ensuring they are as effective as possible. It's like having a custom-fit suit but for your health.

Interactive Element: Reflective Journaling Prompt

To make this journey of discovery more personal:

- Pause for a moment and consider the impact of these

advancements on your own life. Take some time to journal about the gut health challenges you face.

- Visualize how the upcoming technologies and treatments could transform your approach to these challenges.
- Imagine a future where managing your gut health is as straightforward as using a personalized probiotic or receiving daily updates from an intelligent toilet.

This isn't merely a flight of fancy - it's an exercise in bridging the gap between future innovations and your health journey, making the prospect of a healthier gut more authentic and exhilarating.

In closing this exploration of gut health's future, it's vital to acknowledge that every new piece of research, each technological breakthrough, and all emerging therapies contribute to a revolution in our understanding and management of health. From detailed microbiome maps to treatments customized according to our genetic makeup, the future holds endless promise. Remain curious and well-informed and be prepared for the next significant advancement in gut health that could dramatically alter our approach to wellness in unimaginable ways.

10.2 PERSONALIZED NUTRITION AND GUT HEALTH

In the buzzing universe of health and wellness, personalized nutrition emerges as a shining star, promising a tailored approach to your dietary needs based on a trio of crucial factors: your genetic makeup, your unique lifestyle, and the diverse community of microbes residing in your gut. This burgeoning field is akin to having a nutritionist, a geneticist, and a gastroenterologist collaborating in the kitchen to whip up a custom meal plan that sings in harmony with your body's specific requirements. It's about moving away from the one-size-fits-all dietary recommendations to a more nuanced symphony of food choices that resonate perfectly with your individual health needs and goals.

Personalized nutrition isn't just about indulging in your personal food preferences. It dives deep into how your genes interact with various nutrients, how your daily activities influence your nutritional needs, and how the teeming world of bacteria in your gut affects everything from your metabolism to your mood. For instance, while kale might be a superfood for some, for others, it could lead to bloating and discomfort due to variations in gut flora or genetic differences in nutrient absorption. Personalized nutrition decodes this complex interplay, offering diet plans that optimize your gut health and, by extension, your overall well-being.

Implementing this customized approach begins with gathering detailed insights into your body through advanced testing. This could involve genetic tests that reveal how your body metabolizes fats and carbohydrates, mapping out the microbiome to understand its composition and health, or even blood tests that provide snapshots of nutrient levels and inflammatory markers. With this data, nutrition professionals can craft diet plans that precisely meet your nutritional needs and fit seamlessly into your lifestyle, preventing the hit-or-miss outcomes often accompanying standard dietary advice. It's about turning the data from these tests into actionable eating habits that can transform your health and life.

However, tempting as this tailored approach may sound, it comes with its challenges and ethical considerations. One of the primary hurdles is accessibility. Genetic and microbiome testing costs can be prohibitive for many, potentially creating a divide where personalized nutrition becomes a luxury for the few rather than a standard approach for the many. Moreover, privacy concerns exist regarding how personal genetic and health data are stored and used. Ensuring this sensitive information is handled with the utmost confidentiality and protected against misuse is paramount in fostering trust and broader acceptance of personalized nutrition.

Another consideration is the potential for information overload. Interpreting complex genetic data and microbiome analyses isn't straightforward and can sometimes lead to more confusion than clarity. Without the guidance of knowledgeable professionals who can translate this data into practical dietary advice, individuals may make health decisions based on misinterpretations of the data or oversimplified conclusions. This highlights the necessity for a collaborative approach in personalized nutrition, where multidisciplinary teams of healthcare providers work together to ensure that the recommendations are scientifically sound, clinically relevant, and easily integrated into daily life.

As we continue to explore and expand the boundaries of how diet influences health through the lens of personalized nutrition, it becomes clear that this approach can revolutionize how we think about eating and how we manage health and prevent disease. By tailoring nutrition to the individual, we're not just feeding the body - we're nourishing it as efficiently and effectively as possible, paving the way for a future where diet is as personalized as medicine, tailored to each individual's unique genetic and microbial makeup. As this field grows, it promises to bring us closer to the goal of therapy: to treat disease and prevent it, ensuring a healthier, happier future for everyone.

10.3 INTEGRATIVE APPROACHES TO GUT HEALTH

Imagine treating your gut health like you're conducting a symphony. Each section of the orchestra plays a crucial role, and the harmonious integration of strings, winds, brass, and percussion creates a stunning musical experience. Similarly, an integrative approach to gut health combines various therapies and practices, ensuring that physical, mental, and emotional aspects are all tuned to contribute to your overall well- being. This holistic health model isn't just about mixing and matching treatments—it's about orchestrating a personalized wellness strategy that resonates perfectly with your body's needs.

The concept of a holistic health model extends beyond conventional medical treatments to include a range of complementary therapies. These therapies, which include acupuncture, herbal medicine, and various stress reduction techniques, offer a rich palette of options to enhance gut health. Acupuncture, for instance, is not merely about inserting needles into the body at random points - it's based on ancient practices that consider the energy flow, or qi, in the body. For gut health, acupuncture can help regulate digestive functions and alleviate pain and bloating. It's like hitting the right notes to soothe the body's internal rhythms.

Herbal medicine also plays a significant role in this integrative ensemble. Herbs like ginger, peppermint, and turmeric aren't just staples in your spice rack—they're potent remedies that can reduce inflammation, combat nausea, and support digestive health. Imagine brewing a cup of peppermint tea that doesn't just warm your hands but also calms your stomach. These natural ingredients provide gentle yet effective ways to tune your gut health without the harsh side effects that sometimes accompany prescription medications.

Stress reduction techniques like yoga, meditation, and guided relaxation are the percussion section of our orchestra—subtle yet powerful. Chronic stress can throw your digestive system out of rhythm, leading to gut health issues. Integrating stress management practices can help maintain the gut-brain axis, the critical communication link between your digestive system and mental state. By reducing stress, you're smoothing out the wrinkles that disrupt this communication, allowing your gut and brain to sync beautifully.

When considering integrative approaches, the chorus of excitement around their benefits must be tempered with a commitment to evidence-based practice. It's essential to distinguish between what genuinely works and merely anecdotal. Each integrative therapy in your gut health plan should be supported by scientific evidence, ensuring it's safe and effective. This rigorous approach prevents the cacophony of unproven methods from drowning out the beneficial effects of validated therapies. It's about being discerning, choosing only those complementary practices that have been shown to work harmoniously with conventional medical treatments to enhance your gut health.

Personalized treatment plans are the conductors of this integrative orchestra, ensuring that each therapy is introduced at the right moment and tailored to your unique health needs. Just as a conductor adjusts the music's tempo and dynamics to suit a hall's acoustics, a personalized treatment plan considers your specific symptoms, lifestyle, and preferences. This customization might involve tweaking dietary recommendations based on your body's responses, choosing herbal supplements you tolerate well, or scheduling acupuncture sessions to address particularly stressful periods.

Implementing a personalized, integrative approach to gut health allows for a dynamic and flexible management strategy that adjusts to your body's changing needs.

Whether introducing probiotics to aid digestion, using acupuncture to relieve stress- related symptoms, or incorporating herbal remedies for inflammation, each element is selected to support and enhance your gut health concertedly. This holistic strategy addresses immediate symptoms and promotes long-term well-being, ensuring that every aspect of your health is harmonized in a continuous symphony of care.

10.4 NAVIGATING THE WORLD OF GUT HEALTH TESTS

As we explore this intriguing landscape, you'll discover that the tools available— ranging from microbiome analyses to food sensitivity tests—aren't just cool tech gizmos. They're your health detectives, providing clues that help piece together the puzzle of your digestive well-being.

Types of Tests

First, consider microbiome analyses as a detailed survey of your gut's inhabitants. These tests pinpoint the variety and abundance of bacteria within your digestive system, shedding light on the richness of your gut's ecosystem. Next in line are the food sensitivity tests, which assess your body's responses to various foods, helping identify potential dietary triggers. Finally, we delve into digestive function tests, which scrutinize the efficiency of your digestive machinery by evaluating factors such as acid levels and enzyme production.

Interpreting Results

Having these tests is one thing, but understanding the results is another game altogether. Interpreting these results can be as tricky as reading a foreign language without a translator. That's why professional guidance is crucial. It ensures that the insights you gain aren't just random data but meaningful information that can guide your health decisions. For instance, a healthcare professional can suggest specific probiotics or dietary changes if a microbiome analysis shows you're low in a particular beneficial bacteria. Without this expert translation, you might find yourself trying to solve a Rubik's cube in the dark—frustrating and futile.

Test Limitations

However, it's vital to approach these tests with a healthy dose of skepticism. Not all tests are equal, and some limitations could hinder your health quest. For example, some food sensitivity tests might flag a food as a problem based on antibodies your body might not even react to, leading to unnecessary dietary restrictions. Or, a microbiome test might only partially capture the dynamic nature of your gut's bacterial community, which can change daily. Knowing these limitations is like learning the blind spots in your car's mirrors—you can compensate for them by seeking multiple perspectives and getting comprehensive advice.

Integrating into Health Planning

Finally, integrating the findings from these tests into your overall health planning is like using a GPS during a road trip. It's one thing to have a map, but knowing how to use it to navigate effectively is what gets you to your destination. In health terms, this means taking the insights from your gut tests and translating them into actionable steps under the guidance of health professionals. Whether tweaking your diet, adjusting your probiotic intake, or addressing specific digestive issues, these actions are informed by complex data tailored to your body's needs. This strategic integration ensures every adjustment is a calculated step towards better gut health rather than a shot in the dark.

Navigating the world of gut health tests is an exciting journey into the unknown territories of your own body. With the right tools, professional guidance, and a critical mind, you can unearth valuable insights that empower you to take control of your digestive health. Armed with knowledge and supported by science, you're not just passively experiencing your health journey —you're actively directing it, one test result at a time.

10.5 THE ROLE OF FASTING IN GUT HEALTH RESTORATION

No, not the kind where you skip dessert. I'm diving into the type that might reboot your gut health. You've probably heard whispers about fasting everywhere, from fitness blogs to wellness podcasts, painting it as a near-magical solution for everything from weight loss to enhanced mental clarity. But let's strip away the hype and focus on what it can do for your gut. When done right, fasting isn't just a break from eating - it's like hitting the pause button on your digestive system's never-ending playlist of tasks, giving it a precious moment to catch its breath and repair itself.

Fasting Benefits

The benefits of fasting on gut health go beyond just giving your stomach a break. During fasting periods, the reduced workload allows your gut lining, often bombarded by frequent eating, to repair and regenerate. This can lead to enhanced microbiome diversity—imagine it as biodiversity in a rainforest, where a wide variety of species (or, in this case, bacteria) thrive, each contributing to a healthier ecosystem. Moreover, fasting can improve digestive efficiency by allowing your body to focus on absorption and assimilation when you eat rather than constantly processing incoming food.

Types of Fasting

Before you envision a daunting, food-free horizon, let me introduce you to the various types of fasting that are much more approachable than you might think. Intermittent fasting, for example, is like the casual Friday of fasting methods. It's adaptable and relatively easy to integrate into your lifestyle. This method typically involves 16-hour fasting windows daily coupled with 8-hour eating windows, effectively limiting your culinary adventures to a manageable part of the day. Then there's time-restricted eating, which might sound similar but is more like setting a curfew for your stomach. It focuses on consuming all your meals within a specific timeframe each day—say, between 10 a.m. and 6 p.m., which might align better with your body's circadian rhythms, enhancing natural digestion and metabolism.

Scientific Evidence

But let's get real—does science back up the buzz? Absolutely. Numerous studies have tipped their hats to fasting, highlighting its benefits not just for waistlines but for gut health, too. Research shows intermittent fasting can increase beneficial gut bacteria, such as those linked with reduced inflammation and improved bowel function. These changes can contribute to a more substantial intestinal barrier, your gut's first line of defense against toxins and pathogens. Fasting can help fortify your gut's security system, keeping the bad guys out and the good vibes in. The impact of fasting on insulin sensitivity can also play a role in managing blood sugar levels, indirectly supporting gut health by stabilizing the internal environment in which your gut flora operates.

Considerations and Precautions

However, it's not all smooth sailing. Fasting, like any dietary change, comes with its set of considerations and precautions. It's crucial to approach fasting as you would any new exercise regime —gradually and with professional guidance. For those with certain health conditions, such as diabetes or gastrointestinal disorders, or for pregnant women, fasting might require modifications or might not be advisable at all. It's essential to consult with a healthcare provider to tailor fasting methods to your specific health needs and conditions. Hydration is another critical factor. During fasting periods, ensure you're sipping on plenty of water to keep dehydration at bay, as it can be a sneakily everyday sidekick to fasting.

As we explore fasting as a tool for gut health restoration, consider it part of a broader, balanced approach to health. Integrating fasting with a diet rich in nutrients, regular physical activity, and proper sleep creates a holistic health strategy supporting your gut and entire being. Whether you dip your toes into the fasting waters or dive headfirst, understanding its role and potential benefits can equip you with one more strategy in your quest for optimal health. So, as you ponder the idea of giving fasting a go, remember that it's not about deprivation. It's about empowerment —a way to give your gut a breather and boost its function, paving the way to a healthier gut and a happier you.

10.6 BUILDING A LONG-TERM GUT HEALTH MAINTENANCE PLAN

Imagine your gut health as a lovely garden you've worked hard to cultivate and maintain. Just as a garden needs regular watering, weeding, and adjusting to the seasons, your gut health thrives on consistent care and the ability to adapt to changes. Establishing sustainable habits is akin to laying down a well-thought-out blueprint for your garden. It's about finding a routine in your dietary and lifestyle choices that suits your current life and can be adjusted as your needs and circumstances evolve. This might mean setting regular mealtimes that sync with your body's natural rhythms or incorporating various foods to ensure gut microbes get the diverse nutrients they need to thrive.

Sustainability in your gut health regimen also includes recognizing the foods and activities that nourish your body and those that don't. It's about being mindful of how different foods affect your gut and overall health and adjusting your eating habits accordingly. This doesn't mean you need to stick rigidly to a specific diet. Instead, it's about creating a flexible eating pattern that can evolve with your health needs and lifestyle changes. For example, you might need more fiber-rich foods as you age, or certain probiotics help you manage stress better. Keeping this flexibility in mind ensures your gut health plan remains effective and sustainable over the long haul.

Regular monitoring is essential. Just as a gardener regularly checks their plants for signs of distress or disease, keeping a close eye on your gut health symptoms and triggers is crucial. This might involve tracking your dietary intake, noting how different foods affect digestion, or keeping a symptom diary. Regular monitoring allows you to catch potential issues early and adjust your diet or lifestyle before minor symptoms become significant problems. It's also helpful during visits to your healthcare provider, giving you concrete data to discuss and base your health decisions on. But life is full of changes, and your gut health maintenance plan needs to be adaptable. Whether it's a change in your job that alters your stress levels and eating habits, a new phase in your life like pregnancy or menopause, or new scientific findings that shed light on better gut health practices, being open to modifying your approach is critical.

For instance, if you find increased stress at work is causing digestive upset, you might need to incorporate more stress-reduction techniques or adjust your diet to include more gut-soothing foods. The ability to adapt ensures that your gut health strategy remains relevant and practical, no matter what life throws your way.

Incorporating mental and emotional health practices into your gut health plan is also vital. The connection between the gut and the brain means that your mental state can significantly impact your digestive health and vice versa. Practices like meditation, yoga, or even regular social interactions can improve your mental and emotional well- being, which in turn can help maintain a healthy gut. Viewing gut health as part of your overall holistic well-being—not just food and digestion—ensures a more comprehensive approach to health targeting all aspects of your well-being.

In wrapping up this chapter, remember that building a long-term maintenance plan for your gut health is like tending a garden. It requires patience, regular care, adaptability, and a holistic approach that includes your mental and emotional well-being. By establishing sustainable habits, regularly monitoring your health, adapting to changes, and integrating mental health practices, you're setting the stage for a thriving gut that supports your overall health and happiness. As we move forward, let these principles guide you in nurturing a gut health regimen that grows and evolves with you, ensuring a vibrant and flourishing life.

CONCLUSION

I'm reminded of my humble beginnings in this vast universe of gut health. Years ago, as I grappled with the relentless symptoms of Hashimoto's disease, I felt like a passenger in my own body, watching helplessly as it veered off course. The frustration with conventional treatments that barely scratched the surface of my discomfort led me down a path of discovery into the intricate world of gut health. This journey was not just about finding relief - it was about reclaiming my life and vitality.

By sharing my story and the powerful insights I've gained along the way, you, too, can feel empowered to take the reins of your health. Remember, your gut is not just the site of digestion - it's the command center for your overall well-being, influencing everything from your mental clarity to your emotional balance. The scientific evidence is clear: a balanced microbiome is foundational to good health, and neglecting this aspect can lead to many health issues that extend far beyond the stomach.

Throughout this book, we've explored various strategies to nurture and restore gut health—from the foods that feed our microbiome to the lifestyle changes that reduce stress and enhance our digestive efficiency. Each chapter was designed to inform and transform complex scientific concepts into practical, everyday actions to improve your gut health.

Education is power, and understanding the intricacies of your gut health is the first step toward lasting wellness. This book aims to light your path towards a healthier, more vibrant life by demystifying the science and offering clear, actionable advice. But remember, this isn't a sprint, it's a marathon. A journey that requires patience, listening to your body, and being willing to adjust based on what it tells you.

So, what's the next step on this journey? Start simple. Introduce a serving of fermented foods into your daily diet or establish a calming bedtime routine to enhance your sleep quality. Small changes can lead to significant results, and the journey to better gut health begins with a single step.

I also invite you to join the community of fellow gut health warriors. Connect with us through online platforms and social media groups where we share our challenges and celebrate our successes. You're not alone on this journey. There's so much we can learn from each other.

Thank you for allowing me to be a part of your health journey. The strategies and insights shared in this book will improve your gut health and open doors to a life filled with energy, balance, and joy. Here's to a healthier, happier you—inside and out!

THE BEGINNER'S GUIDE TO GUT HEALTH

UNLOCKING DIGESTIVE FREEDOM, WEIGHT WELLNESS, AND MENTAL CLARITY MADE EASY

Simply by leaving your honest opinion of this book on Amazon, you'll show other people wanting to learn more about gut health where they can find the information they're looking for, and pass their passion for gut health forward. Thank you for your help. Gut health is kept alive when we pass on our knowledge – and you're helping me to do just that.

Scan the QR code below to leave your review:

REFERENCES

1. Allen, J. M., & Mailing, L. J. (2018). Exercise Modifies the Gut Microbiota with Positive Health Effects. Integrative Physiology, 8(1), 75. https://doi.org/10.3389/fphys.2017.00157

2. Aurora, N., Bhatia, M., Clapp, M., Herrera, L., Wakefiled, S., Wilen, E., "Gut microbiota's effect on mental health: The gut-brain axis". *National Library of Medicine: National Center for Biotechnology Information.* 2017. https://www.ncbi.nlm.nih.gov/pmc/articles/PMC5641835/

3. Bose, P., Ph.D.. "Leaky gut linked to depressive disorders: New insights into microbiota-induced epigenetic changes". *News: Medical Life Sciences.* 2023. https://www.news-medical.net/news/20231218/Leaky-gut-linked-to-depressive-disorders-New-insights-into-microbiota-induced-epigenetic-changes.aspx

4. Cassata, C. "8 Easy Tips to Avoid a Grumpy Gut While Traveling". *Healthline.com.* 2019. https://www.healthline.com/health-news/how-to-keep-your-gut-healthy-while-traveling

5. Cruzat, V., Macedo Rogero, M., Noel Keane, K., & Curi, R. (2018). The Roles of Glutamine in the Intestine and Its Implication in Intestinal Diseases. International Journal of Molecular Sciences, 19(1), 92. https://doi.org/10.3390/ijms19010092

6. Cryan, J. F., & Dinan, T. G.. "Gut microbiota's effect on mental health: The gut-brain axis". *National Library of Medicine: National Center for Biotechnology Information,* 2017. https://www.ncbi.nlm.nih.gov/pmc/articles/PMC5641835/

7. Cryan, J. F., & Dinan, T. G. (2015). The gut-brain axis: Interactions between enteric microbiota, central and enteric nervous systems. Annals of the New York Academy of Sciences, 1312(1), 9–24. https://doi.org/10.1111/nyas.12669

8. DeAngelis, D. "21 Simple Meal Prep Ideas to Help Support Gut Health". *EatingWell.com.* 2023. https://www.eatingwell.com/gallery/8032015/simple-meal-prep-ideas-for-gut-health/

9. Emmalee. "Helping You Achieve Vibrant And Lasting Health". *Awake & Well: Holistic Health Simplified.* Accessed May 23, 2024. https://awakeandwell.co/

10. Evertz, C. "Nurture Your Gut Health This World Digestive Day". *Martin & Pleasance*. 2023. https://martinandpleasance.ca/blogs/wellness-hub/nurture-your-gut-health-this-world-digestive-day

11. Fallivan, J., M.s., R.D.N.. "Why Is Gut Health So Important? Ask A Nutritionist". *Barrier Islands Free Medical Clinic*. 2023. https://www.bifmc.org/why-is-gut-health-so-important-ask-a-nutritionist/

12. Gentile, C. L., & Weir, T. L. (2021). The association of weight loss with changes in the gut microbiota: A review of the literature. Gastroenterology Research and Practice, 2021, Article ID 9747387. https://doi.org/10.1155/2021/9747387

13. Graf, D., Di Cagno, R., Fåk, F., Flint, H. J., Nyman, M., Saarela, M., ... Jakobsson, H. E. (2021). Contribution of diet to the composition of the human gut microbiota. Microbial Ecology in Health & Disease, 26(1), 26164. https://doi.org/10.3402/mehd.v26.26164

14. Guigoz, Y., & Doré, J.. "Role of prebiotics, probiotics, and synbiotics in management of inflamatory bowel disease: Current perspectives". *National Library of Medicine: National Center for Biotechnology Information*, 2023. https://www.ncbi.nlm.nih.gov/pmc/articles/PMC10130969/

15. Gurney, E. P., & Clish, C. B. (2021). Spotlight on the Gut Microbiome in Menopause. JAMA Network Open, 4(9), e2124723. https://doi.org/10.1001/jamanetworkopen.2021.24723

16. Gut Microbiota For Health. "Gut microbiome in 2023: Current and emerging research trends". *Gutmicrobiotaforhealth.com*. 2023. https://www.gutmicrobiotaforhealth.com/gut-microbiome-in-2023-current-and-emerging-research-trends/

17. Harvard Health Publishing. (n.d.). "The gut-brain connection". *Harvard Health Publishing: Harvard Medical School*. 2023. https://www.health.harvard.edu/diseases-and-conditions/the-gut-brain-connection

18. Harvard T.H. Chan School of Public Health. "The Microbiome". *Harvard T.H. Chan: School of Public Health*. Accessed May 23, 2024. https://www.hsph.harvard.edu/nutritionsource/microbiome/

19. Lin, H., Ou, Y., Wu, L., Yang, T. "The role of probiotics in women's health: An update narrative review." *National Library of Medicine: National Center for Biotechnology Information*. 2024. https://pubmed.ncbi.nlm.nih.gov/38216265/

20. Liu, Y., Song, R., Song, Z., Wu, Z., Zhang, X. "Effects of ultra-processed foods on the microbiota-gut-brain axis: the bread-and-butter issue". *ScienceDirect.com*. 2023. https://www.sciencedirect.com/science/article/abs/pii/S0963996923002752

21. Merotto, L. (n.d.). Why Good Sleep Hygiene is Essential For IBS Freedom and Digestive Health. Retrieved from https://www. leighmerotto.com/blog/how-sleep-affects-ibs-digestive-health

22. National Center for Complementary and Integrative Health. "'Detoxes' and 'Cleanses': What You Need To Know". *NCCIH.NIH.gov.* 2019. https:// www.nccih.nih.gov/health/detoxes-and-cleanses-what-you-need-to-know

23. National Institute of Diabetes and Digestive and Kidney Diseases. "Eating, Diet, & Nutrition for Irritable Bowel Syndrome: How can my diet help treat the symptoms of IBS?". *National Institute of Diabetes and Digestive and Kidney Diseases.* 2017. https://www.niddk.nih.gov/health-information/ digestive-diseases/irritable-bowel-syndrome/eating-diet-nutrition

24. National Institutes of Health: Office of Dietary Supplements. Probiotics: "Fact Sheet for Health Professionals". *National Institutes of Health: Office of Dietary Supplements.* 2023. https://ods.od.nih.gov/factsheets/Probiotics-HealthProfessional/

25. OmegaQuant.. "Vitamin D and Digestion". *Omegaquant.com.* 2023. https://omegaquant.com/vitamin-d-and-digestion/

26. Palsdottir, H., MS. "11 Probiotic Foods That Are Super Healthy". *Healthline.com.* 2023. https://www.healthline.com/nutrition/11-super-healthy-probiotic-foods

27. Pendulum. (n.d.). How Hydration Affects Your Gut Health. Retrieved from https://pendulumlife.com/blogs/news/how-hydration-affects-your-gut-health

28. Rezaie, A., Pimentel, M., & Rao, S. S.. "Small intestinal bacterial overgrowth: Management". *UpToDate.com,* 2024. https://www.uptodate. com/contents/small-intestinal-bacterial-overgrowth-management

29. Selhub, E. "Nutritional Psychiatry: Your brain on food". *Harvard Health Publishing: Harvard Medical School.* 2022. https://www.health.harvard.edu/ blog/nutritional-psychiatry-your-brain-on-food-201511168626

30. Smiley, B. "How Much Fiber Should I Eat Per Day?". *Heathline.com.* 2023. https://www.healthline.com/health/food-nutrition/how-much-fiber-per-day

31. 31. Smith, K. J., & Aitken, R. J. (2023). Do probiotic interventions improve female unexplained infertility? A systematic review and meta-analysis. Reproductive Biomedicine Online. Advanced online publication. https:// doi.org/10.1016/j.rbmo.2023.08.007

32. Sonnenburg, E., Sonnenburg, J. "Fermented-food diet increases microbiome diversity, decreases inflammatory proteins, study finds".

Stanford Medicine: News Center. 2021. https://med.stanford.edu/news/all-news/2021/07/fermented-food-diet-increases-microbiome-diversity-lowers-inflammation

33. Tech, Q. "8 Ways To Boost Your Immune System And Naturally and Fight Off Infections". *Max Health*. 2022. https://www.maxhealthsolutions.com.ng/2022/01/ways-to-boost-your-immune-system.html

34. "The gut-brain connection". *Harvard Health Publishing: Harvard Medical School*. 2023. https://www.health.harvard.edu/diseases-and-conditions/the-gut-brain-connection

35. Tomova, A., Bukovsky, I., Rembert, E., Yonas, W., Alwarith, J., Barnard, N. D., ... Dinan, T. G. (2021). The Gut Microbiome and Female Health. Frontiers in Medicine, 8, 684217. https://doi.org/10.3389/fmed.2021.684217

36. Tri-State Gastroenterology Associates. (n.d.). How Stress Affects the Gut Microbiome. Retrieved from https://tristategastro.net/how-stress-affects-the-gut-microbiome/

37. Valdes, A., Vijay, A. "Role of the gut microbiome in chronic diseases: a narrative review". *National Library of Medicine: National Center for Biotechnology Information*. 2021. https://www.ncbi.nlm.nih.gov/pmc/articles/PMC8477631/

38. Volpe, J., RDN, LD, CLT. "What is a Gut Health Dietitian Nutritionist?" *Whole-isticLiving.com*. 2024. https://wholeisticliving.com/gut-health-dietitian-nutritionist/

39. Wallace, C. J. K., & Milev, R. (2021). Probiotics for the treatment of depression and its comorbidities. Expert Opinion on Biological Therapy, 21(5), 561–573. https://doi.org/10.1080/14712598.2021.1891099

40. Wallace, C., Milev, R. "The effects of probiotics on depressive symptoms in humans: A systematic review". *Annals of General Psychiatry*. 2017. https://doi.org/10.1186/s12991-017-0138-2

41. Wellness, R. "Natural Remedies for Candida Overgrowth". *Rose Wellness Center for Integrative Medicine*. 2024. https://rosewellness.com/natural-remedies-for-candida-overgrowth/

42. William, M. "How Total Health and Fitness Can Improve Your Mental Well-Being". *Nswtrt.org.au*. 2022. https://nswtrt.org.au/how-total-health-and-fitness-can-improve-your-mental-well-being/

43. Zeratsky, K., R.d., L.D.. "What are probiotics and prebiotics?". *Mayo Clinic*. 2022. https://www.mayoclinic.org/healthy-lifestyle/nutrition-and-healthy-eating/expert-answers/probiotics/faq-20058065

44. ZOE. (n.d.). Intermittent Fasting, Gut Health, and Your Microbiome. Retrieved from https://zoe.com/learn/intermittent-fasting-gut-health

Made in the USA
Las Vegas, NV
27 December 2024

15457852R00085